Assessment of the Elderly Patient

Assessment of the Elderly Patient

Second edition

F I Caird DM FRCP
Reader in Geriatric Medicine,
University of Glasgow

T G Judge MB FRCP
Consultant Physician in Geriatric Medicine,
Longmore Hospital, Edinburgh

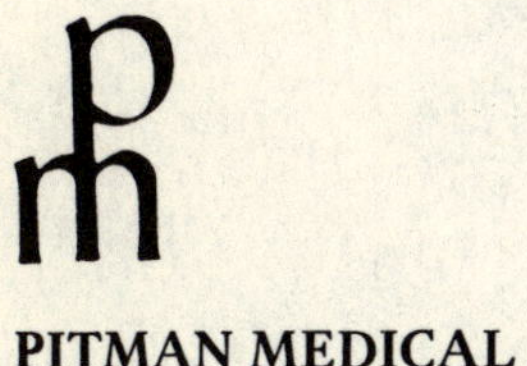

PITMAN MEDICAL

First published 1974
Second edition 1979

Catalogue Number 21 039981

Pitman Medical Publishing Co Ltd
P O Box 7, Tunbridge Wells,
Kent, TN1 1XH, England

Associated Companies

UNITED KINGDOM
Pitman Publishing Ltd, London
Focal Press Ltd, London

CANADA
Copp Clark Pitman, Toronto

USA
Fearon Pitman Publishers Inc, San Francisco
Focal Press Inc, New York

AUSTRALIA
Pitman Publishing Pty Ltd, Melbourne

NEW ZEALAND
Pitman Publishing NZ Ltd, Wellington

British Library Cataloguing in Publication Data

Caird, Francis Irvine
Assessment of the elderly patient. – 2nd ed.
1. Geriatrics 2. Diagnosis
I. Title II. Judge, Thomas Grieve
618.9'7'075 RC953 78-41252

ISBN 0-272-79549-6

Set in 11 on 13 pt. IBM Journal by
Gatehouse Wood Limited, Cowden, Kent
Printed and bound in Great Britain
at The Pitman Press, Bath

Contents

Foreword

by Professor Sir Ferguson Anderson, OBE, CStJ, MD, FRCP,
David Cargill Professor of Geriatric Medicine,
University of Glasgow

The title of this book describes the new approach to the care of old people. This might be summarized in the need for accurate diagnosis made after the use of modern scientific investigation, if such is necessary; the total consideration of the medical, mental and social conditions of the elderly person; and, with compassion and understanding, a plan for comprehensive therapy and continuing treatment.

As a committed believer in this teaching, I am delighted to be writing these few words, as I feel that the many important technical advances in medicine have tended to blind the physician and to conceal the need to keep in mind the essential components of daily life in a dwelling-house. The individual cannot be assessed without knowledge of his home circumstances. In my own unit the custom of the physician to visit the elderly patient in his own home has added a new dimension to the knowledge of the hospital doctor and made him much more aware of the facts of life in the community.

With increasing information about the older ill person, physiological changes have been noted which in turn affect the symptoms and signs of disease. The authors of this text have pointed clearly the way to accurate diagnosis and stressed its importance, but have also directed the reader's thought to the practical aspects of health and disease in the context of the elderly individual's environment.

For me it is an immense pleasure to see this book written by members of my own department. I am naturally proud of their endeavours and utterly convinced of the correctness of their thesis. This text will be of immense help to all concerned with the elderly and more importantly will eventually be of great assistance to older people everywhere.

Preface to First Edition

Although the fact that the medicine of old age is a separate speciality has been recognized from the earliest times, indeed by Galen, it is only within the last 30 years that the full implications of this concept have been recognized.

The first and most important idea is that no one is ill simply because he is old, but because he has a definite and identifiable disease. Once this idea is accepted, many ancient but still current beliefs about senility and ageing must be dismissed. The second and much more recent idea is that every individual must be considered in relation to his environment. Such a concept is old in pediatrics, but is still new and indeed revolutionary with regard to adults. The third concept is that of multiple pathology. The occurrence of multiple disease processes in the same individual is the main clinical characteristic of the older patient. Multiple pathology, however, means more than this. It means the possible coexistence of physical, psychological, nutritional, and social disturbance in the same person. The fourth concept is that, just as the process of growth in childhood may modify disease processes, or indeed complicate them, so the process of ageing may complicate diseases of later life, so that the manifestations of disease in older people are different from those in the young and middle-aged. The most important difference is the frequent lack of specific symptoms, which arises in part from modification of sensory responses. Thus an acute duodenal ulcer may not present with pain, but with vague ill-health. Again it is likely to be difficult to diagnose meningitis in an elderly patient who cannot bend his neck because of cervical spondylosis. Thus multiple pathology makes diagnosis difficult, and the ageing process may complicate the assessment of the sick and elderly patient.

Despite these difficulties it is imperative that accurate diagnosis and complete assessment should be achieved whenever this is possible. Once outdated ideas of senility and ageing are discarded, there is no more rewarding field of medicine than the management of the older patient. Given reasonable assessment the therapeutic possibilities are enormous. Even conditions which are relatively difficult to treat in younger people, such as malignant disease, may behave quite differently in the elderly. The management of superficially more simple conditions such as congestive cardiac failure may be more difficult in the elderly, but can produce very great benefit to the individual patient.

But before treatment must come adequate assessment. It is our purpose in this book to describe how the assessment of the older person differs from that of the younger. We have tried to indicate some of the basic requirements for this assessment, and to point out simple and practical ways in which it can be achieved. The introduction of teaching in the special skills of geriatric medicine into the curricula of many medical schools suggests that there is a need for a simple guide to the assessment of the elderly patient and to the diagnosis of common disorders in old age, which might be of value to the senior medical student, to the newly qualified doctor, and to those in training as general practitioners and physicians. We believe knowledge of these topics to be of great importance, if only because the work of every doctor, whether he be in general practice or in the hospital service, is increasingly concentrated upon the older patient.

There are certain differences between the layout of this book and others dealing with clinical examination and diagnosis. We have chosen to group together discussion of physical signs under the part of the body where they occur, rather than by the body system to which they relate. Thus discussion of the venous pulse will be found in the chapter on the head and neck, and not in that on the cardiovascular system. The chapter on the lower limb includes discussion of disorders of joints, arteries, veins, and of the nervous system as they affect that part. We feel that this is in fact how clinical examination is carried out by clinicians of experience, and that our readers will already have some experience of history-taking and examination of the adult patient, and so be capable of rearranging physical signs in their own minds to give a proper description of each of the body systems.

In the preparation of this book, we have many people to thank. We are indebted firstly to our teachers and colleagues, past and present, who have stimulated our interest in the details of assessment of the elderly patient, and more particularly to those of our colleagues who have been kind enough to read and criticize the manuscript, and offer their valuable suggestions for its improvement: Professor W. Ferguson Anderson, Dr Anne Gilmore, Dr R. Archibald, Dr G.A. Broe, Dr N. Cowan, Dr R. Davidson, Dr I.E. Hughes, Dr J. Thompson and Miss Agnes Crombie, SRN. Any virtues this work may have are due to their suggestions and influence; the defects are our own.

Preface to Second Edition

A second edition must justify itself by incorporating definite and substantial changes from the first. In the present case we can point to removal of factual errors and correction of mistakes of emphasis to be found in the first edition, and more importantly to changes with time in the practice of geriatric medicine and in our own views on a number of issues. Thus the increasing availability of sophisticated investigations for the elderly patient has made it desirable to amplify the chapter on laboratory investigations to bring it into line with present-day practice, and to indicate the knowledge needed for the proper application of such investigations to the problems of the individual sick elderly patient.

The introduction of SI units has not brought with it any greater benefits to geriatrics than to any other branch of medicine; we have attempted to temper the metric wind to the physicianly lamb by giving both traditional and SI units where these differ.

Our own thoughts on the team approach to the assessment of the elderly patient in hospital have been greatly improved and sharpened by experience of the invaluable assistance that can be given by physiotherapists, occupational therapists, and social workers trained, usually by apprenticeship rather than by formal study, to work with the elderly and to appreciate their particular problems and the solutions to them. Other changes have resulted from clearer thinking on the subject of chronic brain failure and on the importance of injudicious drug therapy as a cause of symptoms of old age.

We are as before, heavily indebted to many colleagues for their influence on our ideas and practice, in particular to Dr A.J. Akhtar, Professor W.B. Jennett and Mr G.M. Teasdale. Much of the final chapter is taken from an article in *Medicine* by one of us. We are grateful to the editor and publishers for permission to use material from this article.

Chapter 1
Social Assessment

In all broadly based medical specialities the patient is properly viewed as an individual in relation to an environment. Such an approach is especially relevant in the elderly, since multiple pathology does not mean merely the simultaneous occurrence of numerous disease processes in various systems in the same individual, but also the possible coexistence of physical, psychological, nutritional, and social disorders in the same patient. In addition, geriatricians have come to appreciate that breakdown in any one of these four compartments frequently predisposes to disturbance in the other three. For example, in a recent survey emotional disturbance was found to be less than half as common in healthy old people as in the physically ill.

Historically the need for social assessment of the older patient arose in part from practical necessity. When the geriatric services began, the combination of the very large number of old people awaiting admission, and the lack of available beds, made assessment of priorities essential; consequently home visiting for the purpose of social assessment began. It was soon realized that such assessment had a much wider application than simply the allocation of priority for admission to hospital. Indeed, it is true that if the home has not be examined, the elderly patient has not been properly assessed. Information may be gained from a home visit either directly by the doctor or indirectly by a district nurse or health visitor. This information is of value in several different ways.

Firstly, an assessment of the urgency of the presenting situation may be made. An elderly patient who develops broncho-pneumonia, but who lives in a good home and is surrounded by attentive relatives who know what to do and are prepared to do it, can easily be treated at home in the absence of complications. The same illness occurring in a patient living alone in a poor home and isolated from relatives and friends would demand immediate admission to hospital.

Secondly, factors contributing to the illness can be assessed. A rapid survey will reveal the likelihood of neglect, malnutrition, dehydration, alcoholism, or drug intoxication.

Thirdly, the potential physical barriers to rehabilitation and resettlement at home can be evaluated. Obviously an elderly person who has suffered a recent stroke and lives in a good home without stairs to climb and with an inside toilet, presents an entirely different problem to a person who lives alone up several flights, or has a distant outside toilet.

Fourthly, the relationship between the old person and his relatives or friends can be assessed, and some idea gained of the depth of their feeling for him, and of their willingness and ability to help him. Affection cannot be presumed from physical proximity or close family relationship, and the lack of it could clearly constitute a major psychological barrier to recovery and resettlement.

It is as important to have a system in mind when the home is visited as it is to have a method for examining the cardiovascular system. In neither case must vital facts be overlooked. Such an approach should include consideration of the house itself, the care of the house, the care of the person, the family, and the use of supporting services.

The House

In making an assessment of the house the following points must be considered: the stairs, the toilet and bathing facilities, water supply, cooking arrangements, heating, lighting, ventilation and accident hazards. It is important to distinguish not only between good and bad housing, but also between housing which is appropriate or inappropriate to the individual concerned. Thus a well-kept house reached by means of a difficult flight of stairs may seem at first sight better than a poor home on the ground floor, but may in fact be quite inappropriate if the person who has to live there is frail and has difficulty in climbing stairs. It is essential not only to consider, but actually to see, each room the old person lives in, and all the stairs and steps he may need to negotiate.

Since half or more of elderly people in the community suffer from some degree of restriction of mobility the stairs they have to climb may play a decisive role in their well-being. It is necessary to consider, whether or not the patient is, or ever will be, fit to climb the relevant stairs. If the answer is 'No', then no matter how good the housing may be, it is inappropriate. If the stairs are badly lit, unevenly placed, worn, without a good handrail, or with a poor surface, they may constitute a serious accident risk. Recent city building has tended to favour the multi-storey block of flats; here a lift is an essential part of the way of life, and the frequency with which it breaks down can be a limiting factor in an old person's existence. It is important to find out whether or not the patient can operate a lift, since some elderly people adapt badly to innovations. If the patient cannot use such a lift with ease, there is a very real danger of social isolation.

There is a great variation in the standard of toilet facilities in houses; it is unusual for the elderly to be specially favoured. It is quite possible for a patient to become incontinent of urine solely because he is unable to reach adequate toilet facilities. Many old people are faced with a toilet situated on a flight of stairs, up or down from the living area. Such a toilet may be communal, outside the house, or indeed at the bottom of the garden, and may be quite inaccessible to anyone suffering from a neurological or locomotor disorder. Where an old person can reach such a toilet he may avoid visiting it for as long as possible because of embarrassment, distaste of the state of the toilet itself, or in wintertime dislike of the temperature. It is not surprising that bowel habits may become disordered or that faecal impaction may result. Such toilets rarely have handwashing facilities, with the consequent hazard of cross-infection. The size of the toilet is also of great importance to a disabled person, particularly if a walking aid or wheelchair is used; there must be adequate room to get in and out. Sometimes the provision of a simple aid such as a handrail or grip may make all the difference between recurrent misery and a reasonable existence. It is most unlikely that points such as these will be appreciated by someone who has not visited the home and examined it with due care.

The water supply is also of critical importance to the well-being of elderly people. If there is no water supply in the house at all, then no patient with any substantial degree of disability will be able either to keep clean or cook adequately. If the only inside supply is of cold water, as is still the case in older housing, then the frequent boiling of kettles is necessary. It is often difficult, if not impossible, for disabled people to carry a full kettle, particularly if they require a walking aid. Either they do without hot water or they are exposed to a serious risk of scalding.

There are still many houses which have no bath. It is unrealistic to expect a frail, elderly housebound patient to keep clean under these circumstances. Even where a bath is available many disabled patients who live alone are afraid to use it, lest they find themselves unable to get out of it.

Sometimes this situation can be relieved by the provision of a simple bathing aid such as a grip, a rail, a seat, or a non-slip mat. The occupational therapist is best placed to advise on the appropriate aid. Failing this it is necessary to arrange for supervision of the patient's bathing. Unless there is very severe deformity or disability, such supervision does not require the skill of the already overworked district nurse, but may be carried out by an intelligent and able-bodied relative, friend or help who is trusted by the patient.

Inadequate cooking facilities can add to the consequences of ignorance, apathy, and fixed bad food habits, and result in disorders of nutrition. Even a minimally adequate diet is extremely difficult to obtain if the only cooking appliance is a single gas burner or even an open fire. Any degree of difficulty with locomotion, or any significant impairment of mental function will clearly make such a situation much worse. Again, unless the cooking facilities have been seen, the possibility of malnutrition or sub-nutrition may be missed. At this stage it is often simple to get some idea about the supplies of food in the house and hence of the ability of the individual to look after themselves.

Adequate heating is expensive, and many elderly people living on low incomes heat their houses quite inadequately. Unfortunately the choice may lie between being cold and being hungry. Sometimes the elderly choose another way out of this dilemma and lie in bed for as long as possible wrapped in all the available coverings. Even this may be quite inadequate to protect an elderly person with an unstable heat regulating mechanism from the danger of hypothermia. Where heating is inadequate, ventilation is often restricted in an attempt to conserve existing heat. There is consequently a risk of fire, or even of carbon monoxide poisoning.

Again, when heating and ventilation are unsatisfactory, natural or day lighting is usually poor also. Inadequate lighting, be it natural or artificial, can readily impair or even prevent reading, cleaning and cooking and also increases the chances of accident.

Accident Hazards

Three-quarters of all fatal home accidents in Great Britain occur in people aged 65 and over, and the number of such accidents increases each year. By far the most common cause of fatal home accidents is a fall, with poisoning, and burns and scalds coming next. The morbidity of accidents is much greater than their mortality, since in addition to the discomfort and disability they produce, fear and inactivity frequently follow their occurrence. Not all falls in the elderly are accidental; many follow episodes of disturbed consciousness. One-third of all accidental falls occur on stairs, where the absence of a hand-rail is often a factor. Loose rugs on slippery floors, worn floor coverings, inappropriate footwear, such as ill-fitting soft slippers, and decrepit furniture or fittings create further serious and remediable hazards. Such hazards must of course be assessed in the light of the patient's mental and physical state. It is obvious that what is a mild danger to a healthy person can become a serious risk if brain failure or locomotor instability is present.

Problems with gas fires and cookers are common, partly because of forgetfulness, confusion, and clumsiness, and partly because of failure of the sense of smell. The risk of carbon monoxide poisoning has been reduced by the introduction of natural gas, but fire hazards to the patient and neighbours remain very important. It is essential to use appliances which fail safe, and to encourage the use of fire-guards.

It has been known for many years that barbiturates are contra-indicated in older patients, because they increase confusion and produce postural hypotension; despite this barbiturates are still a common cause of poisoning in the elderly, as are other psychotropic drugs such as anti-depressants and tranquillizers. Alternative hypnotics should always be prescribed in older patients (e.g. triclofos, temazepam, or chlormethiazole), and any potent drug should only be prescribed in small amounts. Furthermore, if on every home visit an enquiry, and if necessary an inspection of cupboards were carried out, the accident hazard to the old, as to the young, of powerful drugs could be reduced.

The Care of the House

So far we have dealt with the house itself, and outlined some of the features which should be carefully looked at in assessing home conditions during a visit to the house. The information to be obtained from studying the way in which the house is looked after requires similar attention. The key questions are:

1. Who does the cleaning?
2. Who does the cooking?
3. Who does the shopping?

If the patient normally does all these things unaided then any illness which affects mobility—and any illness whatsoever may do this in old people—will precipitate a crisis. Such a situation can be resolved only by the provision of attention as a matter of great urgency. Failing this, admission to hospital may be required. If other people carry out these tasks then a similar crisis can arise if they are taken ill or go on holiday.

In the longer term, the accessibility of the shops may be an important consideration, and here there is as ever no substitute for detailed local knowledge, best of all acquired by visiting the house.

The adequacy of these domestic arrangements is of much greater importance than the actual state of the house. It is most important not to have preconceived ideas of cleanliness and tidiness. Obviously rat-infested squalor is totally unacceptable to anyone of any age but an older person who is well and happy in his own home, however unclean and untidy, may well be better off than the same individual miserably clean and regimented. As always the individual and the environment must be considered together.

Difficulty in maintaining the garden as a result of physical or mental disability or lack of help, may be an important consideration in rehousing.

The Care of the Person

In looking at the house, structural difficulties were considered which could give rise to social disabilities. Now we must look at the adequacy of the functional capacity of the patient to care for himself. Again there are several questions which require to be answered, each essentially with two parts—What is the problem? and What is it due to? Here the assistance of an occupational therapist to assess in detail the needs of the patient can be valuable, both in hospital and for the old person at home.

The questions are:

1. Is the patient prevented by disease or disability from feeding unaided? If this is so, immediate action must be taken to prevent dehydration and starvation.
2. Can the patient dress unaided? Again if the answer is 'No', immediate help is required to prevent social disintegration.
3. Can the patient cope with bladder and bowel function? It is important to distinguish true faecal and urinary incontinence from enforced soiling caused by immobility

or disability. Would the provision of a commode solve any existing toilet problems, especially nocturnal ones?

4. Is the patient prevented by disease or disability from dressing her own hair? This is a thoroughly demoralizing situation for any woman and may lead to complete neglect of all other personal care.
5. Can the patient care for the feet without assistance? It must be borne in mind that foot disorders are among the commonest causes of limited mobility in older people in this country at the present time; many result from inability to carry out adequate care unaided, and are easily remediable with the help of a chiropodist.

The Family

Our civilization has moved far from the primitive tribal pattern of family life, and family bonds are looser now than in former generations. The important practical questions to be asked in assessing the importance of the family in the support of a given elderly person are to discover what relatives the patient has, where they live, and what is the strength of the relationship between them and the old person. It is clearly unrealistic to expect relatives to travel long distances to look after an old person who lives alone, or to expect much help from a close relative living nearby who has not spoken to the patient for many years. Periodically reports appear in the newspapers of the bodies of people living alone being found weeks or even months after death. It is only too easy to be critical of the family and friends in such cases, but it is essential to remember that many older people drive relatives and friends away by their behaviour; such behaviour in itself may be a symptom of underlying disease.

Somewhat similar considerations apply to old people living with their families, since even the strongest bonds of affection can be severely damaged by difficult behaviour on the part of the elderly person. Some symptoms give rise to greater stress in the family than others. For example, urinary incontinence is surprisingly well tolerated in a loved one, though faecal incontinence is much less easily accepted. Confusion is often acceptable, whilst loss of sleep, nocturnal wandering and severe curtailment of family social life are not. Apart from this, members of the family and indeed, neighbours and friends may have other important commitments, e.g. the rearing of young children. The competing loyalties which may result are the source of much distress and difficulty. In considering the value of family and community support to the individual, it is essential at the same time to consider the social priorities. We never cease to be impressed by how much the majority of young people do look after and help the elderly, and by the infrequency of the problems of rejection and neglect.

One important practical consideration is the inadvisability of the doctor appearing to take sides in disputes within a family over the care of an old person. These must always be left to the family themselves to resolve as best as they can.

In assessing the isolation or otherwise of an old person it is important to know about the number of relatives and their geographical location, as well as the strength of the relationships. Similar considerations apply to friends and neighbours. It is important to remember that for old people suffering from the effects of social isolation voluntary visiting societies are available. It is unfortunate that some patients who need help in time of trouble are denied pastoral visiting from their church.

Supporting Services

In considering this aspect of the social situation, one must ask three principal questions:

1. What supporting services is the patient receiving?
2. Which services does the patient require?
3. Which services are available in the area in question?

There is considerable local variation both in the availability of various welfare services and the methods whereby they may be deployed to help the patient. Local knowledge is of paramount importance in this connection, and has no substitute. In addition, where payment for services is required, as in the case of home help, it is important to know whether the patient or his relatives can afford the necessary payments, and perhaps more important, whether they are willing to pay for them if they have resources.

The answers to the first two questions presuppose a knowledge of what welfare services in fact exist, and what their functions should be. These may be listed:

1. *The Health Visitor*

Her duties are to visit the elderly and others who are at risk for their health. The health visitor's services are usually activated by the general practitioner, and it is becoming increasingly common for health visitors to be attached to individual practices or group practices. The district nurse may also call upon the health visitor to visit, and so may neighbours and relatives. Her role is to advise on general problems in connection with the health of the elderly, and to put them in touch with the appropriate agencies which can help solve them, in particular with the patient's own general practitioner or with the Social Work Department. She may arrange for home helps, or for 'meals-on-wheels' to be provided. The health visitor provides informed professional advice, acts in an educational role, and may well be a 'case-finder' for a group of doctors. In the future she may well carry out visiting of all people known to be at risk from the 'Age-Sex Register'. Her duties cover not only the elderly, but also child welfare, ante-natal care and the health difficulties of the entire family, including the problem family.

2. *The District Nurse*

Her duties are to nurse the elderly sick, e.g. to do dressings and administer necessary injections, and not to provide for such things as weekly baths, which can be perfectly adequately carried out by less highly trained people, or by voluntary bodies outside the District Nursing Service.* The district nurse is usually sent by the general practitioner, or occasionally by hospital departments, in particular geriatric departments having district nurse attachments, and rarely by anyone else. She reports to the general practitioner or to the hospital, or on occasion when district nurse and health visitor functions are being carried out by the same person, to others. In the future, State Enrolled Nurses working on the district under the supervision of district nurses may well carry out some of these functions, and so relieve the district nurses.

3. *The Social Worker*

The developing role of social workers in the care of the elderly has been considerably accelerated by the setting up of Social Work Departments. The social worker may be called in by the general practitioner, the health visitor, the health department, or the hospital, and assist in problems of rehousing, institutional care, and on occasions the provision of

* There are sometimes problems of acceptance of voluntary workers by professionals. These could be lessened by offering better training facilities to voluntary bodies.

long-stay hospital care. The next few years are bound to see the development of close links between social workers in Social Work Departments and both hospital geriatric departments and general practitioners. It may be that specialist social workers with particular knowledge of the problems of the elderly will evolve. Since by Act of Parliament the Social Work Department has a major responsibility for the mental well-being of the community, the social worker should practise psychosocial case work and therapy.

4. *Home Helps*

These are, after the District Nursing Service, the principal support of many elderly people. Their function is to assist with problems of domestic care, in particular with cleaning, shopping and cooking. Other aspects of care of the home, such as window cleaning, are not part of their duties. They are provided by Social Work Departments, except in some country districts, may be temporary or permanent, are provided for a certain number of hours per day, usually two, and rarely function at weekends. In most areas if there are relatives, in particular younger female relatives, who can assist in the domestic care of the elderly person, after a brief period, usually of about 8 weeks, payment of what seems an unacceptably high rate is demanded. This frequently results in the elderly person not being able, or thinking themselves unable, to accept the Home Help Service. In some areas of the country a family relative may be officially recognized as a home help and receive payment for her services. In future it is hoped to develop a specially skilled cadre of home helps who will carry out additional social and simple nursing duties.

5. *The Meals-on-Wheels Service*

This is a unique example of co-operation between voluntary bodies and statutory local government services. The Meals-on-Wheels Service is run by the WRVS, and should be called in where there are problems of nutrition, particularly from immobility or psychiatric disorder. In theory, home helps should be able to carry out most of the duties of the Meals-on-Wheels Service, in particular, shopping and cooking, so that when a home help has been provided Meals-on-Wheels should not be provided. The general practitioner, the health visitor, and occasionally members of the general public can arrange for Meals-on-Wheels, either via the Social Work Department, or directly through the WRVS itself.

6. *Chiropody*

This may be provided by the Health Service, or privately. The elderly person may attend the chiropodist or he may visit the home. The arrangements by which chiropody may be obtained vary considerably from area to area, but they are usually either private, or may be made through the general practitioner, the health visitor, or the district nurse.

7. *Domiciliary Physiotherapy*

This is probably one of the most underused of all services, and its organization varies very greatly from area to area. Sometimes it can only be arranged through the hospital physiotherapy department, and then often only on the recommendation of a consultant. This makes for considerable difficulty in providing the service at home. In other areas the health authority may have a staff of physiotherapists, and the general practitioner may arrange for physiotherapy at home for his elderly patients through the district medical officer. In other places the service may be directly available through the physiotherapy department of a small hospital, and may then be much more directly available to the general practitioner.

8. *Domiciliary Occupational Therapy*

This service is of great value in the assessment of the needs of the elderly person in his own environment, in deciding on the need for and providing modifications to the home, such as ramps, hand rails, toilet aids, bathing aids etc. Close co-operation between the occupational therapist in the hospital and in the community is of the greatest importance; ideally at least one person should be common to both teams.

9. *Blind Welfare Service*

This is a separate local authority service now under the Social Work Department. There is a statutory duty to register those with sufficient degrees of visual disability (a visual acuity of less than 6/60 in both eyes, or a visual field of less than 10° in both eyes). Registration can only be carried out by an ophthalmologist. The benefits of registration as blind include visiting by the Blind Welfare Service, reduction in radio licence fees, the availability of talking books, etc., and in some places special arrangements for holidays away from home.

If an older person has poor vision, enquiry should be made as to whether he is on the Blind or Partially Sighted Register. Much effort by all concerned may be saved if it transpires that full ophthalmological documentation has already been carried out.

10. *Old People's Clubs and Day Centres*

It is important to distinguish between old people's clubs, where those attending are mobile and use their own transport, and day centres which are for the frail and where transport is usually provided. Both must be distinguished from the day hospital which is run by the hospital service and provides all the facilities of a general hospital without in-patient accommodation. Clubs and centres may be invaluable in providing both meals for elderly people who are able to get out of the house, but cannot easily cook for themselves (such as elderly widowers), and also human contacts for those who might otherwise become isolated. Some are run by local authorities, some are purely voluntary organizations. In both cases direct contact with the club is the usual method of obtaining the service, and any of a wide variety of people may clearly stimulate the old person to make this contact. Some clubs provide transport for a small number of people who are too immobile to make journeys by public transport.

11. *The Red Cross and Other Voluntary Bodies*

These are particularly important in providing such things as aids for the disabled, e.g. commodes, Zimmer walking aids, walking sticks, wheel chairs, low beds and mattresses (often these can be hired), mackintosh sheets for the incontinent and so forth. Local District Nursing Associations may provide these aids, and in some areas hospital geriatric departments will loan out. Direct application to the local Red Cross or District Nursing Association is the best method of obtaining the service.

12. *Structural Alterations*

Structural alteration to houses owned by local authorities is a service provided in some areas. The domiciliary occupational therapist usually decides what is necessary, and the Social Work Department is then approached to finance the appropriate alterations.

13. *Financial Help*

When the individual requires continual attention both by day and night, the attendance allowance is available. The medical requirements are that the person must have been so severely disabled physically or mentally, for at least 6 months, as to need either frequent attention during the day and/or night in connection with bodily functions, or constant supervision to prevent danger. It should be remembered that allowance is payable in respect of patients in approved nursing homes.

The attendance allowance is obtained by direct application to the local office of the Department of Health and Social Security.

Other forms of financial help may be available from local charitable bodies or trade associations, and also to finance for instance holiday relief, for example from the Chest, Heart and Stroke Association.

14. *Other Services*

These include voluntary visiting, which is little used, and possibly little needed. Voluntary visiting is usually organized by the local Old People's Welfare Association. Night sitter services are available in some areas, but have proved extremely difficult to organize. Laundry services for the incontinent also exist in some places, and may be obtained via the general practitioner, the health visitor, or the district nurse.

Summary

The wide range of available services is obvious, and their proper and economic use depends quite clearly on precise assessment of the old person's needs, and detailed knowledge of how each service may be obtained for the individual in question. With the proper use of the available services it is often possible, but only after full social assessment, to maintain the patient in comfort at home. Such action, initiated in the patient's best interest, may however be misguided or even harmful if a full clinical diagnosis is not accurately made. It is folly to provide social palliation for a treatable medical condition, for example, a home help to clean the house for a patient who has become too tired to do this for herself, when the tiredness is due to iron-deficiency anaemia. Care is no substitute for cure.

Chapter 2
History-taking

There are many differences between what is taught in the standard texts and by most clinical teachers about taking the clinical history, and what is practical or desirable in the elderly. The object of taking a clinical history is the same at any age—to assemble as many relevant facts as possible about the patient and his symptoms. The differences lie both in the technique by which the history should be taken in old people, and also in the interpretation which should be put on some of the symptoms elicited.

The principal differences in technique result from the fact that more time, and considerably more patience, is required in taking a history from an older patient. More time is needed because deafness, impairment of memory, confusion, and on occasion confabulation may greatly impede the normal process of question and answer.

If the patient is deaf, then it is extremely important to communicate in a way that is understood. This means looking directly at the patient so that he can see your face and lips, and not raising the voice more than is necessary. Shouting merely accentuates the vowels, which may be perfectly well heard already, and obscures the consonants, which convey important information, and are the sounds which are especially poorly heard. If necessary an old-fashioned speaking tube, or some other device like an electronic communicator, should be used to amplify the sounds so that the patient can understand. Total deafness may necessitate communication entirely in writing. This is an extremely valuable exercise for the history-taker, as he requires immediately to phrase his questions simply and shortly, and only to ask those which are likely to be important. Otherwise time and patience will soon run out.

Questions need to be as simple and straightforward as possible, and so be less open to misinterpretation. It may only be possible to establish that a symptom exists, without being able to discover how long it has been present. The reverse is also a common occurrence; it may be clear that something has been the matter for a fairly definite time, though its nature is not at all clear. It may be impossible to get any further than this, and if this is the case, there is no point in losing patience either with the patient or with oneself. It must be accepted that all the facts that can be collected have been collected.

Confusion and impairment of memory are frequent obstructions to adequate history-taking. Frank confabulation is fortunately uncommon, but if it is present and no other check can be made on the accuracy of the patient's story, then the only method of detecting it is by inherent improbabilities and inconsistencies in the patient's story. Thus a patient who has clearly been bed-ridden for some days may describe long walks taken that morning, or may give two accounts of what has been happening to him over the last few days which do not agree with each other.

The second important difference in technique is that it is almost always necessary in the case of an elderly person who is in the least ill, in the least confused, or shows more than a minimal degree of intellectual impairment, to take a history from some other person. This is almost always a close relative or some other person who has been looking after the patient. If the history has already been obtained from the old person in the presence of the relative, it is tactful to begin talking to the relative by saying that you wish to go over some points of detail in the story and to confirm that you yourself have got correctly in your mind what has been happening. The implication should always be that it is you, rather than the the patient, who is muddled.

Many symptoms which produce no external evidence of their presence are not of course directly susceptible to enquiry through a second person, but it is usually possible to discover, for instance, if the patient has complained spontaneously of a symptom such as chest pain. Other leading symptoms, such as frequency of micturition, incontinence, insomnia, or poor appetite, are much more obtrusive and obvious and can almost always be reliably determined. An impression can also be gained, and amplified by direct questions, of which symptoms the relatives considers the most disturbing and which might therefore constitute a barrier to resettlement at home.

The second group of problems in history-taking is that of interpretation of symptoms. These problems derive from the fact that in elderly people many conditions present with essentially the same symptoms. A large number of illnesses in old people are first manifest when the patient becomes unable to walk and takes to his bed. Often the patient may develop confusion or incontinence, when these symptoms have not been present before. In the first case, it would be most unwise to assume that the disorder causing inability to walk must be in the locomotor system, in the second that there was necessarily some intracranial condition present, or in the third some urinary disease. Any of these symptoms might well be produced by conditions as diverse as pneumonia, myocardial infarction, urinary infection, drug intoxication, or stroke. It follows from this that the standard equiry into the symptoms relating to specific systems must always follow a plan which allows the determination of symptoms which could be derived from all systems. Such a systematic enquiry might follow the plan set out below.

1. General symptoms: anorexia, fatigue, thirst, weight loss.
2. Gastro-intestinal symptoms: vomiting, abdominal pain,

constipation, diarrhoea.
3. Genito-urinary symptoms: frequency, nocturia, dysuria.
4. Cardiorespiratory symptoms: cough, chest pain, shortness of breath, oedema.
5. Locomotor symptoms: pain in the limbs, back, or joints.
6. Cerebral symptoms: confusion, withdrawal, disorder of speech, paralysis, paraesthesiae, fits, headache, falls.

It follows also from the non-specific nature of symptoms in many diseases in old people and from the fact that most, if not all, disabilities are long-standing in old people that it may be more important to determine the duration of symptoms and their sequence, that is the march of events, rather than to determine the precise symptom which has been present.

The answers to such questions as 'How long is it since he has been able to get out of the house?', 'How long is it since she was able to do the shopping by herself?', will be extremely revealing and are usually accurately answered by the patient or by the relatives. It is also of great importance to attempt to determine the speed of any change of state. A previously fit old person who suddenly takes to his bed, or suddenly begins to fall, or suddenly becomes confused, having been previously entirely lucid, is most likely to have some disorder of sudden onset such as an infection or a vascular episode, and is most unlikely on the basis of these symptoms alone to be suffering from a slowly progressive condition such as chronic brain failure or most locomotor disorders. Conversely if the relatives say that the patient has only recently become confused, but further enquiry shows that in fact there has been loss of interest in the surroundings and current affairs over several months or years, any acute process becomes unlikely, and the final diagnosis will usually be one of some progressive condition. It follows also that it may often be as important to determine what the patient's state was before the symptoms bringing him to the doctor's attention developed, as to decide precisely what the present symptoms are.

These then are the principal differences in history-taking as between older patients and younger. They may be summarized as the need for different techniques, in particular for more time and patience, and the need to rely on the evidence of people other than the patient. The non-specificity of many symptoms in old people leads to the concept that determination of change of state may be more important than determination of what particular symptoms are present.

The Past History

The accurate determination of a patient's past history is probably more important in old people than in middle-aged and young patients. This is because older people have had more time for more things to happen to them, and therefore simply have more past medical history. It is important to discover what major illnesses and operations the patient has suffered in the past, and as far as possible what happened during them, since, for instance, confusion occurring during a chest infection 2 to 3 years previously may well represent the first evidence of chronic brain failure now much more apparent.

Records of previous hospital admissions are important, because it is very frequent for patients to be largely or even completely unaware of what illness has taken them to hospital in the past, or what operation has been performed. This is only rarely due to impaired memory on the part of the patient, but much more often to impaired communication on the part of doctors. Previous medical records may well throw light on the duration of present symptoms. Thus it is a very frequent occurrence for a patient to complain of cough of a few weeks' or months' duration only, and then to find in hospital notes taken 10 years previously there was a complaint of cough of 5 to 10 years' duration at that time. Previous hospital records may also contain information such as reports on chest X-rays, blood counts, and electrocardiograms, all of which may be very valuable when compared with the patient's present results. What form of hospital record is obtained may vary from case to case. In many instances the most satisfactory record is a copy of the letter written to the general practitioner at the time of discharge from hospital. This should be in the general practitioner's files, and will usually have the added virtue of containing the hospital record number. This will enable the full hospital records to be obtained very much more quickly than if it is not known. Another useful source of hospital record numbers is the outpatient attendance card. If it has been kept, it should be seen and the number noted. If the hospital record number is not available, the patient's address at the time of the previous admission to hospital should be obtained, since if it is different from the patient's present address, it will be very much more difficult for the records department to find the correct notes. Almost all combinations of christian and surnames are likely to occur more than once in the files of any large hospital, and further evidence of identity is therefore vital. The address at the time of admission is extremely valuable, and the patient's date of birth may also help to prevent confusion. Obtaining past hospital records, particularly in places where there are many hospitals, and patients are therefore likely to have been admitted to several, even in the relatively recent past, may be a matter requiring some persistence and determination. It should not, however, be shirked on that account, because it is almost always a source of extremely valuable information. In many cases investigations previously carried out need not be repeated, and time, money, and inconvenience to the patient are therefore saved. In other instances such vital information as that an abdominal operation was or was not carried out for a neoplasm may be obtained, and an entirely different light thrown on anaemia or an enlarged liver. Diagnosis in elderly people is difficult enough without omitting to obtain information which is available if only the attempt is made to get hold of it.

Family History

The family history is of relatively little importance in the elderly because there are few disorders which are at all common in old age, where the family history is of diagnostic value. Huntington's chorea is an exception. The customary enquiries into whether there are people in the family with tuberculosis, epilepsy, or rheumatic fever are very largely a waste of time. It is more common for the family history to be important in another connection, because it represents the patient's experience of those common diseases which run in families. Thus if an elderly person is diagnosed as having diabetes, not to know that a close relative of the patient had diabetes for many years and ended with serious complications is to fail to obtain information of great value in the management of the new patient. Similarly, refusal to have an operation otherwise indicated, may on occasions result from the patient's knowing of a relative who had a similar operation and died from it. If one does not know this, the refusal is thought to be unreasonable, with consequent acrimony and difficulty in the management of the patient.

The family history may also be important in relation to what can be expected from the individual's relatives in the care of the patient. If they are unfit, it is reasonable to enquire in what way, and to attempt to assess the degree of disability. This is, however, a poor substitute for actually meeting the relatives caring for the patient and assessing the disability directly.

Drug History

All elderly patients should have enquiry made about what drugs they have been taking in the recent past. This includes both drugs prescribed by a doctor and those not prescribed.

Chronic purgative abuse and chronic analgesic abuse are not rare in old people, and may well be relevant to the diagnosis of unexplained potassium depletion or unexplained chronic renal failure. Drugs prescribed by doctors are, however, much more important as a cause of symptoms in elderly people. Every attempt should be made to obtain as precisely as possible an account of what drugs have been taken, and what have been prescribed and not taken. To find out about the latter may well be important, as for instance when a patient's congestive heart failure recurs because he stops taking the drugs prescribed, thinking he is well. It is relatively frequent, despite improvements in the labelling of drug containers, to have considerable difficulty in determining precisely what drugs have been prescribed, and the most satisfactory and rapid method is to obtain one tablet from each bottle in the house, to discover which tablets have been taken, and then to compare the tablets with one of the readily available drug identification charts. Even this may fail, as drugs that have been on the market for some while may still not be on the identification charts. The doses taken should be as accurately determined as possible, while the time relationship between beginning or ending of taking a particular drug and the course of symptoms may clarify the cause of the latter.

It is also important to determine the presence of any known drug allergy—those to aspirin and penicillin being the most frequent—and to put on record the fact of a drug allergy in as large letters and as bright colours as is necessary to reduce to a minimum the considerable hazards of further administration of the drug. Drug allergies are, however, much less important than straightforward drug intoxication as a cause of serious symptoms in the elderly.

Dietary History

It is of great importance to recognize dietary deficiencies in elderly people, but it must be said that there is as yet no reliable and rapid method whereby deficiency other than of the very grossest degree can be identified. Certain simple enquiries are, however, of great value. It is useful to ask how many hot meals the patient has per week, since the fewer these are the less likely nutrition is to be adequate. The amount spent weekly on food is also of use for the same reason. It is sometimes useful to enquire how much is spent on food for pets, for it is by no means rare for elderly people to spend as much or more on their dogs and cats as they do on themselves.

A dietary history should include enquiry into sources of food, whether from relatives coming into the house, neighbours, Meals-on-Wheels, or attendance at clubs for old people where meals are sometimes (but by no means always) provided. It should never be assumed that because an old person is receiving Meals-on-Wheels nutrition must be adequate; all too often one hot meal is divided into two and made to last the rest of the day, or even the next day also.

A search of the house for how much food it contains is likely to be of value only when obvious malnutrition is suspected. If all that can be found is a few crusts and the odd tin, the patient's nutrition in the recent past must have been grossly defective.

If there is any suspicion of defective nutrition, its cause should be investigated. It may result from long standing, indeed almost life-long, dietary fads. It may be the consequence of a diet prescribed by a doctor (often himself long dead) religiously adhered to over many years. It is most commonly due to mental disorder, and simple poverty may contribute. The purpose of these enquiries is to direct attention to the choice of remedy. Those with life-long dietary fads are unlikely to change them merely because a doctor tells them to, but nutrition may be improved by the addition of supplements. Therapeutic diets can be changed without great difficulty, while malnutrition associated with mental disorder is likely to require some form of close supervision and continuing care in the community. Poverty requires the tactful use of Social Security benefits.

Alcoholism is not uncommon in elderly people, thought its frequency is doubtless reduced because pensions are inadequate to provide for alcohol at its present price. There is, however, a very clear association between alcohol intake and dietary inadequacy. If alcoholism is suspected, both the patient and his relatives must be directly asked how much he takes. It must be remembered that the relatives' account, particularly the wife's, is not necessarily more accurate than the patient's.

Chapter 3
General Examination

The effects of multiple pathology make it necessary that each system in an elderly patient should be examined in detail, since each system may be the seat of some important pathological process. The comprehensive and detailed examination necessary must be made on some sort of plan which by becoming a habit ensures that no omissions are made. Such a plan must cover all systems and yet not be unduly tiring for the patient. Nor should the old person's natural modesty, which is as great or greater than that of the young, be subjected to any strain whatever. Examination that is other than gentle is never justified at any age.

General examination of the patient begins with the first impression, which will give evidence of the degree of illness present, and from the alertness and general demeanour of the patient provide important clues to his mental state. There may be signs of neglect, either self-neglect or neglect by relatives, in the unshaven or more often unwashed appearance of the patient.

The Skin

The skin of the elderly patient shows striking changes which are probably genuinely due to ageing. It becomes thinner, particularly over the backs of the hands and forearms, but often not noticeably so over the upper arms, trunk and legs.

It becomes less elastic, and when picked up does not return to its original position with any speed. Loss of skin elasticity is therefore of no value as a sign of salt depletion. The skin often becomes drier, and over the legs may show to a minor degree the fish-scale appearance of ichthyosis. There may be pallor beyond that due to anaemia, or pigmentation, either general or local. The clinical determination of anaemia in the elderly is best done, as in the young, from the appearance of the conjuctiva or from the nail beds, but at any age is an extremely imprecise affair.

Local *pigmentation* may be due to local skin disease such as that accompanying varicose veins, or may be due to prolonged suntanning in those who have worked out of doors all their lives. Generalized pigmentation of the skin is not rare in the elderly but the cause cannot often be precisely stated. If it is known to have been present for many years, the most likely cause would probably be racial. Certainly in some parts of Great Britain gipsy blood is associated with striking generalized pigmentation. If it is known to have developed recently, then one occasional cause is the ectopic-ACTH syndrome accompanying bronchogenic carcinoma. Other causes such as Addison's disease, chronic liver disease, or malabsorption are all decidedly rare.

The presence of *scratch marks* should be noted, since in the absence of jaundice these may indicate either the relatively common condition of 'senile' pruritus, or the more easily remedied one of scabies. The burrows of the *Acaris* should be looked for in the usual sites, between the fingers and on the palmar aspects of the wrists. Intertrigo under the breasts, in the groins, or under pendulous folds of abdominal fat is another and immediately obvious cause of pruritus.

Senile warts or hyperkeratoses are very frequent. They are raised flat brown or black warty areas, often oval in shape, with the long axis along the line of the skin creases, and found on the trunk and also on the head and neck. These lesions have no significance, and are unimportant except that cosmetically unsightly lesions may require treatment, and that they require to be distinguished from more sinister lesions such as rodent ulcer and epithelioma.

Ordinary *bruises* indicate the likelihood of recent falls, and their presence should be recorded in the case notes, if only to forestall complaints of ill-treatment in hospital. The characteristic sheet haemorrhages of scurvy should not be mistaken for ordinary bruises; they are seen on the backs of the thighs and calves, and may pass unnoticed if the patient is not turned onto his side or face. Haemorrhage into the calf may be mistaken for venous thrombosis, since there is swelling, pain, and tenderness, but in venous thrombosis the blood is confined to the blood vessels. Extensive sheet haemorrhages over the lower legs and feet may trap the unwary into diagnosing gangrene, but then the feet are cold.

The state of the *pressure areas* (buttocks, sacrum, trochanters, knees, and heels) should always be noted in any old person who has been in bed for more than a day or two, because the earliest pressure lesions (reddening of the skin) require prompt treatment if skin necrosis and the prolonged misery of a frank pressure sore are to be avoided.

The hair on the head should be looked at for its texture and, in those whose circumstances make them likely, for lice. The altered texture of the hair may provide a clue to hypothyroidism. The hair on the feet should be noted, as its presence is good evidence against ischaemia of any severity. The hair on the trunk is the best place to look for the characteristic changes of Vitamin C deficiency. The individual hairs are irregular, curlicue, or corkscrew in shape, and the ends are often broken. The follicles are surrounded by small areas of brownish keratosis. These phenomena (Royston's sign) may precede the appearance of scorbutic haemorrhages.

Examiniation of the breasts should never be omitted in elderly women. The atrophy of normal breast tissue makes any lumps more easily felt, and since cystic mastopathia is not frequent in old age, any clearly palpable lump is likely to be malignant. Fixation to skin or muscle should be sought in the usual way, and axillary nodes palpated, in any patient with a lump.

Temperature

The temperature should be recorded in the mouth, or, if the patient is restless, more conveniently in the axilla. The normal mouth or axillary temperature is the same in the elderly as in the young, and fever has the same significance also. But two important points must always be borne in mind. The first is that the absence of fever in an elderly patient does not exclude the possibility of an infection or other condition which might be expected to cause fever. This is particularly true of the low-grade bronchopneumonia so frequent and so often the final illness in the old. The second point is to remember the frequency of hypothermia in old age. This may occur in any severe illness (e.g. stroke, severe infection, or haemorrhage), as a consequence of administration of phenothiazines, in hypothyroidism, and spontaneously in old people who have a persistent defect of temperature regulation, usually due to neurological disease. The diagnosis of accidental hypothermia should not be missed, since when the body temperature falls all parts of the body, including those normally warm because they are covered, such as the skin of the trunk, become cold to touch. The oral or axillary temperature will usually be recorded as 35°C (95°F) which is as low as ordinary clinical thermometers read. Whenever such a temperature is recorded, the true body temperature should be taken *at once* with a low-reading thermometer in the rectum. This procedure should be a reflex in all doctors and nurses. If the rectal temperature is found to be between 32 and 35°C (90 and 95°F) the hypothermia is mild, and all that needs to be done is to prevent a further fall. Under 32°C (90°F) hypothermia is significant and serious.

Chapter 4
Respiratory System

Respiratory diseases are of great frequency and importance in the elderly, both as a cause of chronic disability and of acute illness. Their diagnosis depends even more on accurate clinical observation in the elderly than in the young, because of the limitations of radiology in the elderly, and the impracticability and difficulty of interpretation of many tests of respiratory function. As is the case with other systems, the interpretation and elucidation of symptoms and signs in the respiratory system in the elderly present some important differences from what is commonly taught in textbooks of medicine.

In any detailed history of respiratory disease in an old person, five points require consideration. These are the smoking history, cough, breathlessness, chest pain, and a variety of symptoms which are less frequently enquired after but are often important, such as wheezing, and the effect of weather on the chest.

A proper *smoking history* requires determination not only of what the patient is smoking at present, but what he has smoked in the past. It is frequently useful to enquire about the largest number of cigarettes per day that has been smoked for any long period. This will be frequently much more than is smoked at present, often for the same reason as alcohol consumption is reduced in old age, that income falls on retirement. The age at which smoking commenced is also of some importance. It is useful to remember that the present generation of men in their eighties is the first that has smoked cigarettes for their entire adult lives. It is remarkable how often men of this age began to smoke heavily in the trenches in France in the First World War. An accurate smoking history enables attention to be focused on the age of onset of the cardinal symptom of chronic bronchitis, cough. *Cough* or *sputum* produced every day for 3 months or more in the year for 3 or more years in succession indicates chronic bronchitis, and the early stages are often taken to be those of a smoker's cough, as indeed they usually are. The early stages of chronic bronchitis are usually apparent well before the onset of old age, so that it is useful to enquire how long the patient has had a smoker's cough. The patient should also be asked whether he brings up phlegm from the chest, for many patients who deny cough will admit to producing phlegm, which they must of course have coughed up. Denial of cough is therefore no bar to the diagnosis of chronic bronchitis, since persistent production of phlegm has the same significance. Periods of worse cough, often following head colds, usually during the winter, should also be noted, and some idea gained of their duration, whether for a few days, a few weeks, or several months, as this may have a bearing on the question of prophylactic chemotherapy.

Table 1. Grades of Dyspnoea

1. Short of breath hurrying on level or walking up hills or stairs.
2. Short of breath walking on level with people of the same age.
3. Short of breath walking on the level at own pace.
4. Short of breath on washing or dressing.
5. Short of breath while sitting quietly.

The analysis and classification of *breathlessness* in old people presents some difficulties. The simple grading system set out in Table 1 can be useful even though many old people without evident cardiac or respiratory disease admit to breathlessness on hurrying on the level or on going uphill, and despite the high frequency of other causes of limitation of exercise tolerance, such as obesity, arthritis, and neurological disease. Nevertheless the distance the patient can manage on the flat without stopping, at a reasonable pace, is a good index of the severity of breathlessness. Recent deterioration and, in particular, the development of breathlessness during dressing, walking to the toilet, or even on talking in bed, can usually be easily established. Note should be made of the occurrence of nocturnal dyspnoea and orthopnoea, as these usually (but not always) indicate a cardiac element in breathlessness. Denial of breathlessness or replacement of breathlessness by fatigue as a major symptom seems to be considerably more common in elderly patients with heart disease than in those whose breathlessness is due to respiratory disease. In an elderly patient with respiratory disease the recent onset of extreme fatigue usually signifies not the worsening of respiratory function, but the onset of an acute infection.

Just as cardiac pain is frequently less severe in elderly than in young patients (see p. 38), *pleuritic pain* is not unduly common in the elderly. In particular basal broncho-pneumonia in bed-ridden elderly patients is rarely or never accompanied by pain. There are several possible reasons for this phenomenon. In some cases confusion accompanying an acute chest infection may blunt the appreciation of pain, in others perhaps there may be no true pleurisy, but as with cardiac pain there seems little doubt that some entirely lucid elderly patients with pleurisy do not have as much pain as would be expected. It follows that the absence of pleuritic pain should never prevent a diagnosis of pneumonia. Other causes of chest pain worse on respiration and lateral in site are not infrequent in old age. The pain of a rib fracture, whether traumatic, due to coughing, or pathological, can be very intense.

A number of *other symptoms* less often enquired into are of value in the diagnosis of chest disease in elderly subjects. Many old people with chronic bronchitis complain of wheezing, which may vary from week to week with inter-current exacerbation of their infection, but does not usually vary greatly from day to day or hour to hour. It is frequently worse in winter, but when present does not usually disturb sleep. In this it contrasts with the episodic wheezing of asthma, which tends to vary from day to day, and when present frequently disturbs sleep. Many bronchitics, but relatively few patients without bronchitis complain, of the effect of weather on the chest. When the weather is cold, damp, or foggy, their cough worsens, and they may become more breathless. The presence of these symptoms contributes to the diagnosis of chronic bronchitis.

Clinical Examination of the Respiratory System

This has probably more to offer in the elderly than in the young, partly because lesions causing symptoms in old people are usually substantially larger and so give rise to physical signs, and partly because of the limitations of radiology in the elderly.

Examination of the respiratory system begins with observations on the presence of *cough,* and on the mechanism of coughing. As already mentioned patients may deny having a cough, yet while the history is being taken or they are being examined, they may cough and produce phlegm repeatedly. The strength of cough should be noted since a weak cough implies a substantially greater hazard of serious trouble from a respiratory infection. In addition many ill, weak, and confused elderly patients may not be able to cough, although they have large quantities of pus in their bronchi.

In addition to the observation of the presence and pattern of coughing, the *sputum* should be observed. This is probably the most important single physical sign in the respiratory system. If the sputum is mucoid, there is no severe current infection. Haemoptysis indicates bronchial ulceration or damage to alveoli. Blood-stained mucoid sputum is frequently due to pulmonary infarction, while blood-stained purulent sputum may be due to bronchial carcinoma, or simply to chronic bronchitis.

The *pattern of respiration* should be observed. Periodic respiration of Cheyne-Stokes type is characteristic of dyspnoea of cardiac rather than respiratory origin. Prolonged expiration and rapid inspiration is characteristic of severe airways obstruction.

Most of the standard physical signs in the chest bear the same interpretation in the elderly as in the young. One exception is that deviation of the trachea from a central position may be due to upper dorsal scoliosis. Expansion of the chest is frequently very limited in the elderly, and the use of a tape measure in this connection is valueless except as a test of observer error. Localized restriction of movement is usually present with large lesions in the chest, while impairment of percussion similarly indicates the presence of underlying consolidation or effusion. The auscultatory signs of respiratory disease are frequently somewhat difficult to elicit in the elderly because they may be unable to take the necessary deep and frequent breaths to order. However, bronchial breathing still implies consolidation, and râles not cleared by coughing alveolar exudate.

Chapter 5
Cardiovascular System

Cardiac disease is very common in old age, and a proper interpretation of the history and physical signs pertaining to the cardiovascular system is therefore of great importance. The fact that the treatment of cardiac disease involves the use of powerful and potentially dangerous drugs increases both the benefits of correct and the hazards of incorrect diagnosis.

Proper interpretation of the major symptoms of cardiac disease is particularly difficult in the elderly, since two important symptoms—cardiac pain and dyspnoea—are frequently modified, and a third—oedema—is only relatively infrequently due to cardiac disease.

Cardiac pain in the elderly differs from that in younger patients in that in the former it is frequently very much less severe, though its site and its radiation are identical. This reduction in severity is true both of the persistent pain of cardiac infarction and of the exertional pain of angina. The pain of cardiac infarction may be overshadowed by other principal presenting symptoms such as dyspnoea, confusion or weakness, while the pain of angina may be merely represented by a relatively slight feeling of tightness in the chest, such that the patient may think it scarcely worth mentioning. Why this is so is far from clear. In some instances there is little doubt that it is the presence of other more urgent symptoms that push pain into the background, but entirely lucid old people without other major symptoms may not infrequently have very little pain from cardiac infarction.

Any chest pain, however apparently trivial, should thus be taken seriously in an elderly person, and more emphasis should be placed on the accompaniments of the pain than on its severity. The radiation of cardiac pain is often identical to that commonly observed in the young. The occurrence of angina on exercise, and its relatively rapid relief, within 10 to 15 min at the outside, by cessation of exercise, will enable a proper diagnosis to be made even when the pain itself is relatively slight. It may even indeed be absent, when it is replaced by the simple necessity to stop walking for a brief period.

Dyspnoea of cardiac origin in elderly patients may also be much modified, so that the principal symptom complained of is extreme fatigue. However, paroxysmal nocturnal dyspnoea with orthopnoea remains largely unaffected, in the sense that a clear story can be obtained of waking in the night and needing to sit up. Cough is a frequent symptom of pulmonary congestion in the elderly, and needs to be distinguished from that of bronchitis. The latter is almost always part of a history going back many years, or is associated with a recent head cold, while the cough of pulmonary congestion is almost always of relatively recent onset.

The problems of the diagnosis of oedema are discussed on p. 95.

One further symptom which is occasionally of cardiac origin is *syncope* (see p. 57). This may be due to the sudden cessation of cardiac output accompanying a Stokes-Adams attack, or more rarely to the presence of severe aortic stenosis. In the latter case syncope is usually associated with exertion; the mechanism seems to be failure of increase of cardiac output with exertion, vasodilatation in muscle, and consequent fall in blood pressure.

It is clear therefore that considerable care needs to be taken with the history of cardiac disease in the elderly. The same applies, perhaps with even more force, to the clinical examination of the cardiovascular system. Yet clinical examination is much more likely to provide answers to important practical clinical questions than any assessment which relies heavily on radiology or electrocardiography (see pp. 123 and 124). These investigations often either confirm what is already known from the clinical examination, or tend to confuse the issue by introducing irrelevancies.

Examination of the Cardiovascular System

This begins with determination of peripheral blood flow from the temperature of the hands (see p. 79) and the detection of cyanosis (see pp. 75 and 79).

The *pulse* should be taken at the wrist in the usual way, but there is little or no point in attempting to determine the presence or absence of sclerosis of the radial arteries. If present it is of the Mönckeberg type and bears no relation to occlusive vascular disease elsewhere in the body. The locomotor brachial artery is common in old age, and should not arouse comment, since all it signifies is increased length of the artery. If valvular disease is suspected, the form of the arterial pulse wave is best determined by palpation of the brachial arteries, since these are larger and easier to feel than the radial, and the detection of abnormality is thus easier. The increased rigidity of the arterial wall which is probably a genuine part of the ageing process modifies the form of the arterial pulse, making the upstroke in particular more rapid. This may result in a normal form of arterial pulse in quite severe aortic stenosis. The collapsing pulse of aortic incompetence can be detected relatively easily, and if present signifies severe involvement of the aortic valve. Simultaneous palpation of the brachial and femoral arteries to detect delayed femoral pulsation should not be omitted in elderly patients with high blood pressure. Coarctation of the aorta does in fact occasionally occur in old age, and will be most easily detected by this simple test.

The determination of *cardiac rate and rhythm* from the pulse is carried out in the same way as in the young. Slow regular rhythm may be missed if particular attention is not paid to precise counting of pulse rate over periods as long as half a minute. Such slow heart rates may be the clue to Stokes-Adams attacks as a cause of episodic loss of consciousness. Rapid regular rhythms in old age are commonly due to supraventricular or ventricular tachycardia, or to sinus tachycardia accompanying infections. Irregularities of rhythm are frequent in the elderly. Many old people show infrequent ectopic beats, and these may be ignored. It may be difficult to distinguish frequent ectopic beats from rhythm disorders such as atrial fibrillation, but careful attention to palpation of the pulse and to the venous pulse in the neck (see p. 63) will frequently enable a correct diagnosis to be made. However, in any uncertainty an electrocardiogram should be carried out. This is particularly important in patients receiving digitalis, since the irregularity of rhythm may represent a toxic effect rather than a failure of drug action.

The *arterial blood pressure* continues to provide some of the most important clinical problems in the medicine of old age. These problems are of two kinds, and result mostly from the widespread failure to recognize on the one hand the true normal limits of blood pressure in the elderly, and on the other the very considerable frequency of postural hypotension in old age. Neglect of the normal range of blood pressure in the elderly leads to many old people being unnecessarily treated with drugs of high potency to relieve symptoms attributed to high blood pressure, while neglect of the second problem leads to many incorrect diagnoses of cerebrovascular insufficiency.

Table 2. Useful Absolute Upper Limits of Blood Pressure in Old Age (mm Hg)

	Men		*Women*	
Age	*Systolic*	*Diastolic*	*Systolic*	*Diastolic*
60–69	195	100	200	110
70–79	195	105	210	110
80+	195	105	210	115

Blood pressure levels in elderly people who are well and have no evidence of damage to their hearts or vascular systems from high blood pressure are given in Table 2. It will be seen that the normal upper limit of systolic blood pressure rises to 210–220 mm Hg in women over 80, and diastolic pressures up to 115 mm Hg are acceptable at the same age. Acceptance of these figures demands that elderly patients with blood pressures lower than this level should not be considered as having high blood pressure, should not have symptoms attributed to their blood pressure, and should not be treated for high blood pressure.

The blood pressure should always be recorded both lying and standing in any complete assessment of an elderly patient. In about 10 per cent of fit elderly people the systolic blood pressure will be found to drop more than 30 mm Hg, though it is relatively rare for the standing systolic blood pressure to fall to a level likely to give rise to symptoms (i.e. to under 100–110 mm Hg). Any febrile illness, and a very wide range of commonly prescribed drugs (Table 3) can result in postural hypotension, which is frequently severe enough to give rise to gross symptoms. The patient becomes grey and collapsed when sitting in a chair or standing up or occasionally after walking a few yards, and is found to have a blood pressure usually well below 100 mg Hg. If postural hypotension is suggested by a story of dizziness on sitting or standing, it is wise to take the blood pressure first lying down. If the systolic pressure is below 140 mm Hg or so, the blood pressure should then be taken sitting, either with the legs horizontal or with the legs over the side of the bed, before standing the patient up. Almost all patients whose systolic blood pressures drop to low levels on standing will show a substantial though smaller drop on sitting, and the embarrassment of having rapidly to return a collapsed old person to the horizontal can be anticipated and avoided.

Table 3. Drugs Commonly Causing Postural Hypotension

Antihypertensives
Benzodiazepines
Diuretics
Levodopa
Phenothiazines
Tricyclic antidepressants

The position of the *cardiac apex* should be determined in the usual way, but it is frequently not clearly palpable. Kyphoscoliosis is very common in the elderly, and if at all marked may result in displacement of the cardiac apex, so that it becomes useless as evidence of cardiac size. It is important therefore not only to note the position of the apex, but also the nature of the cardiac impulse. Left ventricular hypertrophy can usually be reasonably reliably detected from the presence of a powerful and sustained impulse, left ventricular dilatation from a diffuse impulse, and left atrial hypertrophy from a prominent presystolic component before the main outward movement of the left ventricle. Clinical evidence of right ventricular hypertrophy is rare in the elderly, since all causes of right ventricular hypertrophy are uncommon except pulmonary heart disease, and then the hypertrophied right ventricle is almost always obscured by the over-inflated lungs of airways obstruction.

Auscultation of the heart plays an important part in cardiac diagnosis in the elderly, though elderly people frequently cannot carry out the respiratory manoeuvres necessary for a detailed evaluation of auscultatory findings.

The most important points are to determine the presence and nature of *gallop rhythm* and to evaluate the significance of any murmurs present. Normal heart sounds in the elderly are identical to those in the young. Respiratory variation in splitting of the second heart sound is similarly normal, with an increase in the gap between the aortic and pulmonary components during inspiration. If reversed splitting of the second sound is heard, with a narrower gap during inspiration than during expiration, then one of three disorders of left ventricular function is present. These are:

1. left ventricular strain due to hypertension or aortic valve disease;
2. diminution in left ventricular contractility, usually due to recent major cardiac infarction; or
3. delay in left ventricular systole due to left bundle branch block.

A third heart sound (or ventricular gallop sound) is always abnormal, and when heard coming from the left side of the heart, when it is best audible at the cardiac apex, and on occasions may show accentuation during expiration, implies left ventricular failure. A right-sided third heart sound, usually heard in the epigastrium, or the left of the sternum, and very frequently showing marked inspiratory accentuation, is similarly a sign of right ventricular failure. A clinically audible fourth heart sound or atrial gallop is similarly always abnormal, signifying ventricular abnormality, but not necessarily failure. Gallop rhythm may therefore be an important clue to the presence of heart failure or ventricular abnormality as a cause of dyspnoea.

Some phonocardiographic studies have suggested that systolic *murmurs* are present in 60 per cent or more of elderly people. They may or may not be significant. Diastolic murmurs are always significant, as at any age, though the functional importance of the lesions they indicate is of course variable. The common systolic murmur in the elderly is of ejection type, and is heard at the base of the heart, though frequently as clearly at the apex, and is relatively soft (grades 1/4 or 2/6 at the loudest). Such murmurs are thought to be due to minor sclerotic changes at the bases of the aortic valve cusps, giving rise to undue turbulence but not to obstruction or ejection. When a murmur of this type is heard, aortic stenosis should not be diagnosed and the best term is probably aortic valvular sclerosis. In aortic stenosis the murmur is almost always louder and longer, and there is some evidence of left ventricular hypertrophy, either clinical in a substained cardiac impulse, radiological, or electrocardiographic.

Systolic regurgitant murmurs are not rare in the elderly, and may derive from either the tricuspid or the mitral valve. Tricuspid regurgitant murmurs are pansystolic in type, are usually best heard to the left of the sternum in the third and fourth interspaces, usually show striking accentuation during inspiration, and are almost always accompanied by a prominent systolic wave in the venous pulse. This murmur is almost always due to functional tricuspid regurgitation occurring in cardiac failure of whatever cause. Mitral regurgitant murmurs have the same characteristics in the elderly as in the young. They are best heard at the apex, radiate to the axilla, and may on occasion show accentuation during expiration. They are also pansystolic or late systolic in time. When a mitral regurgitant murmur is accompanied by a diastolic murmur or a prominent third heart sound it is safe to diagnose rheumatic mitral valve disease, but when no such signs of mitral obstruction are present, the cause may be either mitral valve prolapse (floppy valve syndrome) or damage to a papillary muscle by cardiac ischaemia.

Pulmonary ejection murmurs are very rarely heard in the elderly, and may for practical purposes be ignored. Their only common cause is atrial septal defect, which in the elderly is accompanied by considerable cardiac enlargement, substantial and fixed splitting of the second heart sound, and a characteristic X-ray appearance, with gross dilatation of the main pulmonary arteries.

A diastolic forward flow murmur in an old person is almost always that of mitral stenosis. An opening snap is not infrequently heard at the onset of the diastolic murmur. The murmur of tricuspid stenosis is very rarely heard in old people, because this lesion is almost always part of severe rheumatic heart disease, which is likely to be fatal in middle-age.

Early diastolic murmurs in old people almost always come from the aortic valve, though the occasional case of pulmonary regurgitation accompanying severe pulmonary hypertension in pulmonary heart disease may be encountered. The aortic diastolic murmur in elderly people is heard in the usual sites, at the base, down the left sternal edge, and at the apex, and is brought out by the usual manoeuvre of leaning forward in expiration.

The proper diagnosis of *cardiac failure* is essential. It is all too common for this to be diagnosed as an obese patient who is breathless and has some ankle oedema due to immobility or varicose veins. Such patients may be treated with powerful and possibly dangerous remedies such as digitalis and diuretics, and do not benefit from them. The contrary error of diagnosing bronchitis in a patient with left ventricular failure will lead to treatment with antibiotics rather than with digitalis and diuretics, and the patient again does not benefit. If the following simple rules are remembered, these errors will be avoided. Congestive cardiac failure should be diagnosed when all of the following five phenomena are present: dyspnoea, elevation of the venous pressure in all phases of respiration, bilateral basal râles, enlargement of the liver (see p. 50) and bilateral symmetrical ankle oedema. If all these five signs are present, then the patient has congestive cardiac failure. If one is absent the diagnosis is unlikely. Left heart failure is less susceptible to precise diagnostic rules, but should be considered when there is dyspnoea, orthopnoea, or paroxysmal nocturnal dyspnoea, together with evidence of a left-sided cardiac lesion, such as left ventricular hypertrophy or dilatation, gallop rhythm, or the murmurs of aortic or mitral valve disease.

Chapter 6
Gastro-intestinal System

Although the symptoms and signs of disease of the gastro-intestinal tract are essentially similar in old age to those commonly encountered in younger people, difficulty frequently arises from the fact that, in the elderly, such symptoms are often due to disturbances outside the gastro-intestinal system. This is especially true of anorexia, constipation, and diarrhoea, which are often leading symptoms of systemic infections, organic brain disease, and psychological or social disorders. Episodes of diarrhoea alternating with episodes of constipation may be as sinister in the elderly as in younger people, but diarrhoea in old age is often spurious, and the result of faecal impaction.

Since pain sensation is diminished in the elderly, major gastro-intestinal lesions may occur without classical symptoms, and diagnosis may be extremely difficult. This is especially true where occult gastro-intestinal bleeding, from for example an asymptomatic hiatus hernia, causes confusion or fainting attacks.

When an older person complains of *loss of appetite*, the most important point to establish is the duration of the symptom. If it is of a few days duration in an old person who previously ate well, a systemic infection or an acute gastro-intestinal disorder is likely; a gradual onset over weeks or months suggests the possibility of a peptic ulcer, neoplasm of the gut or elsewhere, or depressive illness. It is sometimes useful to enquire whether anorexia has been a prominent feature of previous illnesses, since in particular the pattern of symptoms of a depressive illness in a given individual may repeat itself. The usual enquiry into which foods are disliked is of less value in the older patient for two reasons. Firstly, many people as they get older become intolerant of fat and restrict their fat intake; secondly some older people have bizarre dietary habits which are not related to disease.

Difficulty in swallowing is an extremely important symptom at any age. As with anorexia, its duration is the most useful clue to its cause, since dysphagia of more than a few months duration is more likely to be benign than malignant in origin. Difficulty in swallowing first solids then fluids is more likely to be due to malignant obstruction. Nonetheless dysphagia must be considered within the frame of reference of the patient as a whole, since when it is associated with slowness in eating, choking, spluttering, and dysarthria, it is almost certainly neurological in origin and is due to a brain stem disorder, or bilateral hemisphere disease.

Abdominal pain is often difficult to assess in the elderly, partly because of altered pain sensation and partly because of the inability to describe accurately either the principal site of pain or its time relations. Despite the absence of these two crucial diagnostic clues it is usually possible to find out how long the pain has been present in terms of days, months, or years. Occasionally some idea of the organ responsible may be gained from the history. If the pain is related to food or associated with vomiting the origin is more likely to be in the stomach or the small bowel, whereas if it is relieved by defaecation or associated with altered bowel habit then it is more likely to arise from the large bowel. The site of abdominal tenderness is usually much more reliable in locating the site of pain than any description given by an elderly patient.

Assessment of a complaint of *change in bowel habit* is more difficult in the elderly especially if the common obsession with the bowels is present. A long-standing complaint of constipation is thus rarely significant, but a complaint of diarrhoea requires serious attention once abuse of purgatives or the side effects of drugs such as iron and antibiotics have been excluded. As we have pointed out earlier, alternating diarrhoea and constipation may have the same significance as in the young or may be due to faecal impaction. It is important to remember that diarrhoea and constipation may result from systemic disease, for example disorders of thyroid function, as well as from local lesions in the bowel. Psychological factors must also be considered since depression is frequently associated with constipation.

Faecal incontinence is a most distressing symptom in the sentient patient where it may complicate severe diarrhoea or faecal impaction. The latter may be associated with retention of urine and overflow. In the patient with gross mental impairment there may be incontinence even of formed stools, which is almost always accompanied by incontinence of urine.

Examination of the Abdomen

Abdominal examination in the elderly present few important differences from that taught for younger patients. It is often made easier by a thin and lax abdominal wall, or more difficult by obesity. A palpable spleen or other mass has the same significance at any age, but it is important to remember that patients with airways obstruction, large lungs, and low diaphragms may have a liver that is easily felt 1 – 2 cm below the right costal margin. It is smooth, and not tender, and can be shown to be of normal size by percussion of its upper border in the midclavicular line. The kidneys are only very rarely palpable in the elderly, and indeed only quite large renal masses, due to hydronephrosis, neoplasm, or rarely to polycystic disease, can be felt.

One occasional source of difficulty is *pulsation in the*

epigastrium. When this is high up, immediately beneath the xiphoid, and clearly anterior, there is usually no doubt that it originates in the right ventricle; the patient commonly has airways obstruction. When it is lower and posterior, it is important to distinguish between an unusually easily palpable but normal aorta and the potentially lethal condition of abdominal aortic aneurysm. Attention to two points will usually enable the differentiation to be made. If the width of the pulsatile swelling is estimated by placing a finger and thumb on either side of it, and allowance is made for the thickness of the abdominal wall, the normal aorta does not feel more than 2.5 cm or at most 3 cm wide, while an aneurysm is substantially wider. Secondly, auscultation over an aneurysm usually reveals a bruit which can be traced down along the line of both common iliac arteries to the femoral arteries at the groin.

The femoral arteries should be felt when the hernial orifices are being palpated. Neither examination should ever be omitted, nor should rectal examination, which is of great importance especially in sick old people. Failure to carry out rectal examination may leave carcinoma of the rectum or faecal impaction undiagnosed and therefore untreated. It is convenient at the time of rectal examination to test the withdrawn finger cot for the presence of occult blood.

The customary symptoms and signs of *acute abdominal emergencies* may be modified in old people. In general both symptoms and signs tend to be less obtrusive, and are therefore more likely to be overlooked. In particular true rigidity is comparatively rare as a manifestation of peritoneal irritation, and is often replaced by distension. This may be because the relatively weak abdominal muscles are incapable of becoming palpably rigid, and the bowel distension accompanying peritonitis is able to produce striking distension of the abdominal wall. Local tenderness, rebound tenderness, and absence of bowel sounds retain their usual significance, while the occasional patient will show striking local cutaneous hyperaesthesia instead of tenderness.

Chapter 7
Genito-urinary System

Urinary symptoms are very common in the elderly, and two in particular, nocturnal frequency and incontinence of urine, are extremely important as major causes of disability. Incontinence of urine is indeed a prime cause of the need for continuing care in hospital. Most symptoms referable to the urinary tract can be analysed relatively simply if attention is paid to elementary points in the history and examination, and it is important to separate out in particular those cases of incontinence which will repay detailed investigation and energetic treatment.

Frequency of micturition may be associated with the passage of small volumes of urine, when an irritative lesion is likely, or with large volumes; such polyuria is usually due to unregulated diabetes or to chronic renal failure. Similarly a reduced urine volume due to developing cardiac failure must be distinguished from retention of urine. Nocturnal frequency may need particular enquiry, since many old men think it normal to rise twice or more at night, and the loss of sleep and the disturbance of the household is accepted as part of 'normal' ageing. Enquiry should also be made about the amounts of tea, coffee, and other fluids taken late in the evening; their diuretic action is as great in the old as in the young, and surprising improvement may follow their restriction. Similarly the time at which diuretics are given should receive attention in relation to their duration of action, since short-acting diuretics given in the morning do not usually give rise to undue frequency at night, while longer acting drugs, such as some thiazides and in particular chlorthalidone, may still be producing an effect during the night.

Dysuria usually signifies urinary infection in either sex, but many important infections are quite asymptomatic, so that the absence of pain is no guarantee of the absence of infection.

Haematuria may be due to benign or malignant disease of the prostate, or to a bladder tumour, stone, or infection; it always requires urological assessment (see p. 8).

If there is *incontinence of urine*, it is very important to go into considerable detail about the circumstances under which it occurs. Difficulty in handling a urinal may result in a wet bed, but the action needed is clearly not the same as when there is true incontinence.

In old men, incontinence accompanied by frequency and difficulty in initiating and ending micturition is usually due to prostatic disease, often with chronic retention and overflow. If the recent onset of dysuria is mentioned, an infection is likely, though even quite gross infections are, as mentioned, often unaccompanied by pain. When incontinence develops during an acute illness or when constipation is also complained of, faecal impaction will often be found. If none of these symptoms are present, and the old man is incontinent without having any awareness of the desire to pass urine, organic brain disease is very likely, and full neurological examination and simple psychometric testing are necessary. It is also important to enquire whether the patient has any warning of the desire to micturate, since incontinence may be due to locomotor difficulty and failure to reach the toilet in time, rather than to brain disease.

Examination

Palpation of the bladder is the most important part of abdominal examination in relation to the urinary tract. In elderly men with acute retention a tense bladder can usually be felt except in the very fat, and suprapubic tenderness and intensification of the desire to pass urine by pressure over the bladder are of assistance when the bladder cannot be felt. A large lax bladder associated with chronic retention of urine may however be very difficult to feel, and dullness to percussion in the midline above the symphysis pubis may be the only way by which it can be detected.

In old men the external genitalia should be examined in particular for phimosis, and for testicular swellings and hydrocoele. Rectal examination is essential for the assessment of prostatic size, and the detection of the eminently treatable condition of carcinoma of the prostate. The tone of the rectal sphincter may perhaps bear some relation to that of the vesical sphincter.

In elderly women an enlarged bladder resulting from neurological disease or faecal impaction may need to be distinguished from an ovarian or uterine tumour. An ovarian mass usually arises asymmetrically out of the pelvis, and a uterine mass is harder and frequently nodular. In cases of difficulty the enlarged bladder is the only swelling which disappears following catheterization. Retention with overflow in women can sometimes be diagnosed when the bladder cannot be felt, by asking the patient to stand; incontinence follows. In old women rectal examination will assist in the diagnosis of pelvic masses.

Vaginal examination is necessary in elderly women with retention, incontinence, vaginal bleeding, and vaginal discharge. In the nulliparous patient only a single finger examination is possible or humane; it is unusual to gain significant information from such an examination. Normally in elderly women the vagina is atrophic, the cervix is rarely palpable in the absence of polypi or carcinoma, and the uterus and adnexae cannot usually be felt. Vaginal bleeding may require further investigation whether or not vaginal examination is negative, to exclude for example endometrial carcinoma. Vaginal discharge requires bacteriological assessment before the appropriate antibiotic is used along with oestrogen pessaries.

Examination of the urine should never be omitted. Detailed suggestions will be found on pp. 121 and 122.

Chapter 8
Nervous System: History-taking

There are more differences in the examination and assessment of the nervous system in the elderly from that taught for young and middle-aged patients than is the case with any other system. There are three main reasons for this. The first is that there are a number of common abnormalities of the nervous system in the elderly which are of little significance in themselves, yet need to be taken account of in evaluating neurological disorder; the commonest example is perhaps diminution or absence of the ankle jerks. The second reason is the limitation frequently imposed on detailed examination, particularly of sensation, by problems of communication and co-operation in the elderly. The third is that the objectives of neurological diagnosis in the elderly are somewhat more extensive than frequently needs to be the case in the young. Thus it is important not only to make an accurate diagnosis of the pathological process and localization of a neurological lesion, but also to gain an insight into the precise nature of the functional disability produced by the lesion. This is of especial importance in attempting to assess the contribution of a neurological lesion to the patient's disability, when other possible causes are evident, and also in the diagnosis of sensory disorders in patients with stroke, because the existence of such disorders greatly complicates the task of rehabilitation, and their recognition may lead to a much better functional result.

In essence, the neurological history provides evidence of the nature of the process at work in the nervous system, while the examination provides evidence of its location. This is as true in the elderly as at any age, though there are of course exceptions: focal fits may indicate the site of a cortical lesion, and paraesthesiae that of a root lesion.

An episode of neurological disorder that comes on suddenly is likely to be vascular or epileptic in nature, whereas one which progresses slowly over weeks or months is more likely to be a degenerative or neoplastic condition. There are of course, many exceptions to this broad generalization, since episodic deterioration may occur in the course of progressive, degenerative conditions, and also in neoplasm. Nevertheless particular attention should always be paid when taking a history from the patient or his relative to establishing, as precisely as is possible in the circumstances, the true time scale and march of events in any neurological disorder.

It is convenient at this point to consider certain individual symptoms of neurological disorder, such as episodes of loss of consciousness, dizziness, falls, headaches, and paralysis. More specific symptoms, such as those of visual loss and of difficulty with speech or in walking, will be considered elsewhere.

Elderly people not infrequently give histories from which an episodic disorder of neurological function can be inferred. The terms 'dizziness' and 'faintness' are often used, and may refer to extremely varied symptoms. The distinction between true vertigo, faintness, and other sensations is often best achieved by establishing three important points: the circumstances under which the episode occurred, its duration, and whether there was any evidence of true loss of consciousness.

If the episodes only occur on getting out of bed or standing up out of a chair, so that the patient feels faint or blacks out on standing and rapidly recovers on lying, a postural drop in blood pressure is very likely at least a major contributory factor. Such postural light-headedness, or syncope, may occur spontaneously, especially after periods of bed rest, and is also a characteristic and important side effect of many drugs, in particular of all hypotensive agents, of the phenothiazines, and of many other drugs acting on the nervous system, such as the tricyclic anti-depressants. If the attacks occur on moving the head, as on looking upwards to get something down from a high shelf, or on turning the head while walking, either positional vertigo or some condition affecting the circulation in the neck is possible. If they occur under neither of these circumstances, but with the patient either walking, or at rest in bed or in a chair, some other condition (usually cardiac) must head the list of probabilities. Faintness occurring on exertion may also be due to hypotensive drugs, especially to guanethidine and related compounds, and also occurs on aortic stenosis.

If the episodes are only momentary, an extracranial vascular disturbance is usually responsible, if they last for a few minutes a fit or transient ischaemia, if for longer than 5 to 10 min a post-ictal disturbance or, again, transient ischaemia. If they last for longer than 24 hr, structural damage to the nervous system, most commonly of course a cerebral infarct, is probable.

It is frequently difficult to establish whether there has or has not been loss of consciousness, unless a reliable and perceptive witness has been present during an attack. Then it is possible to ask whether the patient seemed aware of what was going on around them, or whether communication with them was quite impossible. Other features of the attack, in particular the presence of paralysis or convulsions, should also be enquired into. The presence of pallor during an attack and, often more strikingly, of generalized flushing during recovery, is highly suggestive of Stokes-Adams disease, in which there is no residual localized weakness as in a stroke, although confusion may persist for varying periods after a single attack, or for long periods when the cardiac output is greatly reduced by bradycardia. Pallor and prolonged subsequent confusion may also accompany a syncopal episode during which the patient was kept upright and the brain thus subjected to prolonged generalized ischaemia.

If there is only the patient's word to go on, then again it is possible to enquire whether he was at all times aware of what others were saying to him, and of what was in front of his eyes. One characteristic type of attack not infrequent in the elderly is the true drop attack, in which the patient suddenly and without warning feels his knees giving way, while he is standing or walking, and falls to the ground. Consciousness is not lost, but the patient is unable to get to his feet again unless he can get his feet against some hard surface to press on, as for instance a wall. There is clearly a sudden failure of maintenance of posture; this is sometimes attributed to vertebrobasilar insufficiency.

It must be admitted that it is often impossible to discover from the history what in fact is the precise nature of 'turns', or 'blackouts', or 'falls'. Under these circumstances an attempt to demonstrate possible mechanisms, such as a postural drop in blood pressure, should be undertaken, the patient should be observed while walking, and if necessary a period of hospital observation arranged in an attempt to provide witnesses for the symptoms.

It is always extremely important to take most seriously a history of *falls* coming on suddenly and without clear cause in an elderly person. An occasional fall clearly due to tripping or some other minor accident may go without investigation, but repeated falls or falls occurring without clear cause are always an indication that a full history and examination of an elderly person is necessary. Nevertheless, especially in those over 75, no definite cause may be found for repeated falls. Loss of postural stability and ataxia of gait may perhaps be due to ageing processes in the nervous system.

Headache is a relatively infrequent leading symptom in the elderly patient, but when it occurs, the most important single fact to be established is its duration. Headache that has been a frequent complaint over many years is most unlikely to have any sinister cause, whereas the new appearance of this symptom in a person not usually subject to headache is likely to indicate at least some new physical or psychiatric condition. The description of the character of the headache retains its importance as in younger people. Elderly patients with headache of functional origin describe pressure on the vertex and tight bands around the head just as younger patients do. The site of the pain is also of some value, since purely occipital headache is a not infrequent manifestation of severe cervical spondylosis, and the pain of ophthalmic herpes and post-herpetic neuralgia is strictly unilateral, and maximum around and above one orbit. Severe headache of sudden onset may indicate the presence of intracranial haemorrhage or meningitis, but in the elderly it is very common for these conditions to produce rapid clouding of consciousness, and the existence of headache may not be apparent.

The presence of local scalp tenderness is a very important symptom of a remediable condition demanding early diagnosis, giant cell arteritis. One of its manifestations is not infrequently severe head pain. It is thus worth enquiring whether the patient has noticed particular tenderness of the head when it is put on a pillow or when the hair is brushed.

Facial pain is again not unduly common in elderly patients, perhaps because few have any teeth, and sinusitis is relatively infrequent. One important cause of facial pain is trigeminal neuralgia, where the paroxysmal nature of the pain, and the frequent existence of trigger areas are usually sufficient to give a diagnosis by themselves.

When a history of *disorder of function of a limb* is given, it must be remembered that the complaint will very likely be the same whether the eventual cause turns out to be predominantly motor, or sensory, or a disorder of co-ordination, or of joint function. The complaint will be of difficulty with walking or with one leg, difficulty with sitting or getting out of bed, or difficulty or clumsiness in the use of a hand. In general pain will suggest a disorder of bones or joints, and its absence a neurological disorder, though root pain from the cervical or lumbar spine, paraesthesiae from nerve compression, and spontaneous ('thalamic') pain are examples of exceptions to this generalization. Nevertheless time is probably better spent on detailed examination of the function of the limb than in taking a history of the precise nature of the disorder of function. The latter is likely to be uncertain and possibly inaccurate. As far as the history goes, the time relations and the severity of the disorder of function are by far the most important facts to establish, together with the pattern of involvement. Thus if there is weakness of one hand, it is very important to know whether there has at any time been weakness of one leg, or whether drooping of one corner of the mouth has been noticed, or any disorder of speech. The simultaneous occurrence of involvement of the face, the hand, and the leg, points to a cerebral lesion probably in the carotid territory, whereas if only one is involved clearly the lesion might well be elsewhere. Similarly the pattern of simultaneous occurrence of difficulty with vision, diplopia, inco-ordination of a hand, and difficulty with walking can be used to locate an ischaemic episode to the territory of the vertebrobasilar system.

Chapter 9
Head and Neck

Examination of the head and neck begins most conveniently with inspection and palpation of the *skull.* Note should be taken of the lateral expansion of the skull in Paget's disease, of the presence of any bony lumps, and of any scars. When the possibility of giant cell arteritis has been raised, local areas of redness or tenderness of the scalp should be looked for, both above and below the hairline, together with the presence of thickness and pulsation in the superficial temporal arteries.

Passive neck movements can then be conveniently tested for. It must be remembered that cervical spondylosis is sufficiently frequent and severe in many old people for them to be unable to get their chins on to their chests. Genuine neck stiffness due to meningeal irritation may thus be difficult to detect on occasion, but when it is present the neck is usually extremely stiff and completely immobile in the sagittal plane, while lateral movement is relatively free. Other signs of meningeal irritation, such as Kernig's and Brudzinzski's, may also be present. Rigidity of the neck in all planes may occur in Parkinsonism, and in patients with evidence of bilateral pyramidal tract disorder.

The neck may then be palpated for abnormal lymph nodes and for thyroid enlargement, and the arterial pulses and venous pressure and pulse examined. The tonsillar lymph nodes may occasionally be felt in elderly people when they are calcified as a result of old tuberculous disease, but these smooth hard and non-tender nodes are the only ones which can ever be considered other than abnormal and sinister in an elderly person.

The same is not true of nodes in the axillae or in the groins. Here small firm mobile nodes are not infrequent, in the axillae probably representing the reaction to injuries and sepsis in the skin of the hands, and in the groins to minor trauma and infection in the feet and legs.

The thyroid is not usually palpable in the elderly, in whom the frequency of goitre varies very much from region to region, presumably with the prevalence of iodine deficiency in childhood and at puberty. The diagnosis of a goitre thus follows the usual rules, which include in particular the determination of consistency of the lump, and a search for evidence of over- or under-function of the gland.

The signs of hyperthyroidism are much less clearly defined than in the young and tend in the elderly to be concentrated in the nervous and cardiovascular systems, with little or no ocular manifestations. Agitation, restlessness, a warm skin, tachycardia, often with atrial fibrillation, and rapid relaxation of the reflexes should be looked for, while lid lag and retraction and exophthalmos are unusual.

The signs of hypothyroidism are similarly somewhat different in the elderly from those taught as characteristic in middle age, and this seems particularly so in men. The skin is dry, but may not be obviously coarse and thickened. Loss of the outer eyebrows is not rare in normal old women, but coarse head hair and loss of the normal regular arrangement of the eyelashes are seen in hypothyroid patients of any age. More attention should be paid to the slow cerebration, husky voice (though this again can be difficult to distinguish from normality), and most importantly, to slowly relaxing reflexes.

The *venous pressure* is in many ways a more important sign to establish correctly than the arterial, because it is the key to the proper diagnosis of congestive heart failure. Two points are important. The first is the not infrequent finding of unilateral elevation of the left jugular pressure and pulse, which may be several centimetres above the right. This phenomenon is due to pressure, mainly during systole, by an elongated aortic arch upon the left innominate vein. If the patient takes a deep breath in, the pressure in the two jugular systems equalizes, probably because inspiration results in movement of the aorta away from the innominate vein. It is important therefore that the venous pressure should be noted during inspiration, and that that in the right side of the neck should be taken.

The second point is that patients with severe airways obstruction may show elevation of the venous pressure in expiration only, as the venous pressure follows the intrathoracic pressure. Again the pressure should be noted during inspiration.

The venous pulse can usually be identified without undue difficulty in the elderly, as the neck veins are easy to see as a result of atrophy of subcutaneous fat and thinness of the overlying skin, though severe dyspnoea or restlessness may prevent proper analysis. The double venous wave of sinus rhythm, the single wave of atrial fibrillation, and the cannon waves of atrioventricular dissociation can usually be seen, and can be helpful in the bedside diagnosis of arrhythmias.

The presence of *arterial bruits* in the neck should be sought for, though when found there may be doubt as to their significance. Arterial bruits may be confused with murmurs transmitted up the large vessels from the heart. The following simple rules will enable the distinction to be clearly made in virtually every case. If the bruit is transmitted from the heart, there will be a basal ejection murmur, usually loud; the bruit will be heard over both carotids and will tend to diminish gradually in intensity as the stethoscope is moved up the neck. In addition the second heart sound will be clearly audible in the neck; only if the aortic component of the second sound is absent (as in severe aortic stenosis) will this not be true. Arterial bruits deriving from carotid stenosis are often, but by no means always, unilateral. They become louder as one goes further up the neck, because they originate almost always from narrowing of the carotid artery at the carotid sinus. The second heart sound will not be audible in the upper part of the neck. There may well be no cardiac bruit. It is also of value to listen over the posterior triangle in the region of the trapezius, for bruits deriving from the origins of the vertebral arteries.

After examination of the neck, it is convenient to begin the examination of the *cranial nerves.* It is rarely necessary to examine the sense of smell in elderly patients, but it may be remembered that progressive loss of sense of smell is in fact very common in the elderly. It is a contributory cause of accidents due to domestic gas and fire, which are less easily appreciated by old people.

The Eye

Examination of the eye is an extremely important part of the assessment of the elderly patient. While no person of whatever age with substantial impairment of vision should be denied the benefit of expert ophthalmological advice, nevertheless physicians caring for elderly people should expect to be able to recognize the commoner diseases of the eye, and be able to make reasonably precise assessments of them. The important symptoms needing enquiry are the duration of difficulty with vision, whether it came on suddenly or gradually, and whether in one or both eyes. The true duration of these symptoms may be difficult to establish, because all patients, and especially the elderly, tend to shorten the duration of ocular symptoms and to maintain that vision has deteriorated 'recently', when in fact it may have been failing, at least in one eye, for years. It is of course normal for elderly people to require glasses to correct presbyopia, and examination and perhaps a change in spectacles is usually needed every three to five years. Changes in vision occurring more rapidly than this, or uncorrectable by spectacles, should at once arouse suspicion. Sudden loss of vision almost always signifies a retinal vein thrombosis or a retinal artery occlusion. Pain and watering should also be enquired about.

Examination of the eye begins with the *eyelids.* Ectropion and entropion are common in the elderly, are causes of considerable irritation and discomfort, and are easily correctable by a relatively simple operation. The *cornea* should be inspected for nebulae, and for small corneal ulcers. These are not rare in old age, and are usually due to trichiasis. There is often no complaint until an inflamed red eye is present, probably because in old age the pain which causes younger patients to seek attention is reduced or absent. Arcus senilis is of no significance whatsoever in the elderly. *The iris* in the elderly frequently shows 'degenerative' changes, by which is meant irregularity of density of pigmentation, and frequently replacement of the normal pigment by palish brown areas. *The pupil* in the elderly is frequently somewhat smaller than in younger people, and may be slightly irregular, but the reactions to light and to accommodation are maintained. Gross irregularity is usually due to synechiae, or on rare occasions to tabes dorsalis.

The *visual acuity* should be measured with whatever accuracy is possible. If formal Snellen type is not available then the headlines of a newspaper may be used to test for lower visual acuities, and the smallest print for higher levels. Determination of finger counting, of detection of hand movements, and of perception of light should be used in the usual way for those with very severe visual impairment. *The visual fields* may be examined by the usual method of confrontation, but in unco-operative patients the menace technique should be used. It is important that the hand should not be brought towards the eye in such a way that a draught of air is set up, and eye closure initiated by a corneal reflex, rather than by a true reaction to menace.

In patients with a left hemiplegia, the condition of left-sided spatial neglect should always be looked for, as its presence constitutes an important barrier to recovery. It is effected by the two pencil test which is done as follows:

Hold two pencils of different colours a foot apart before the patient. Ask him What do you see? If he sees both, change them in front of him; if he can still see both, or indicates by looking to the left, that he knows there is something in his left half-field, significant spatial neglect can be excluded. If he fails to detect the pencil on his left, and is still unaware of it when the two pencils are changed, significant spatial neglect is present.

It should be remembered that it may be dangerous to dilate the pupils in an old person. If the anterior chamber seems shallow or the lens swollen, or if there is any history of episodes of blurred vision, mydriatics should never be used, but ophthalmological advice should be sought. The danger of producing acute closed-angle glaucoma in the elderly is very real.

It is convenient to begin *ophthalmoscopic examination* by examining the lens through a +12 to +15 lens, and slowly decreasing the positivity until the retina is seen. Gross lens opacities will be immediately apparent; it is a relatively simple rule that if the examiner has difficulty in seeing into the eye, the patient may have difficulty in seeing out. Both peripheral wedge-shaped opacities and cobweb-like central opacities are common in the elderly. Peripheral opacities do not in general interfere with vision because they are peripheral, but central opacities will cause a variable degree of visual impairment. The best visual acuity obtained through a pinhole (literally a pinhole in a cardboard disc) can provide useful information. If vision improves to normal or near normal, the visual pathway as far as the retina is intact, and there are no pathological obstructions in the media, even though visualization by the examiner may be difficult.

Examination of the retina by the ophthalmoscope should be systematic. The optic disc, the retinal vessels, the macula, and the peripheral retina should be looked at in turn. The appearances of the optic disc in the elderly are identical to those in younger people. Abnormal degrees of cupping of the disc should be easy to recognize, but if there is any doubt, expert advice should be sought, as the diagnosis of the relatively common and important condition of glaucoma should not be missed. Care should, however, be taken with the diagnosis of cupping of the disc in high myopes, when confusion may result from myopic expansion of the disc.

Papilloedema is very rare in the elderly with intracranial space occupying lesions, probably in part because the frequent simultaneous occurrence of cortical atrophy allows for considerably more space in the cranium to be taken up before the intracranial pressure rises substantially. Papilloedema due to high blood pressure is virtually never seen in patients over seventy. The absence of papilloedema is therefore no evidence of the absence of an expanding intracranial lesion, or of severe hypertension.

Minor abnormalities of the retinal vessels may be ignored in the elderly, since silver wire changes, minor irregularities of calibre, and increase in tortuosity are almost universal in the elderly whatever their blood pressure. It does not greatly advance knowledge of the individual to label these changes as arteriosclerotic. Nevertheless, nipping of the veins at arterio-venous crossings, and the change known as 'banking', where the distal vein is larger in calibre than the proximal, do imply sclerosis of the retinal arterioles, and may on occasion be taken as evidence that the patient's blood pressure is doing him harm.

The physician should be familiar with the four common retinal appearances associated with severe visual impairment in old people. Two of them are usually included together as 'senile macular lesions' or 'degeneration'. In one variety there is deposition of small areas of black pigment in and around the macula. The degree of pigmentation and the degree of visual impairment do not go hand in hand, so that gross ophthalmoscopic changes may be seen with nearly normal vision, and relatively minor degrees of pigmentation may be associated with gross degrees of visual loss. In the second variety there are haemorrhages in and around the macula, some of them deep to the retina. Visual impairment is usually severe.

The other two common retinal disorders are myopic chorioretinal degeneration, and diabetic retinopathy. In the former there is myopic expansion of the optic disc, associated with large areas of retinal degeneration, the white choroid and its blood vessels being clearly visible through the thinned or absent retina. The whitish areas often have margins that are arcs of circles. The changes occur throughout the posterior pole, and may be seen at all ages. In the opthalmological examination of high myopes it is often useful to use a plano lens in the ophthalmoscope and look through the patient's glasses. Diabetic retinopathy in the elderly is almost always of the exudative type. There are aggregated whitish or yellowish exudates at or around the macula, accompanied by microaneurysms and occasional small haemorrhages.

One further important if relatively uncommon occular condition should not escape detection. If an elderly man complains of failing vision, but has no apparent abnormality of the cornea, lens, vitreous, or retina he may well have tobacco amblyopia. The importance of this condition is due to the fact that it is remediable. Almost all patients with it are heavy pipe smokers, but it does occur, if very rarely, in heavy cigarette smokers.

It is next convenient to examine the *eye movements.* This is carried out in the usual way, and in unco-operative patients simply to ask them to look at the examiner standing on one side and then for him to move across to the other side may be sufficient to demonstrate the full range at least of lateral eye movements, and to show up gross nystagmus if present.

The range of eye movements in the elderly is usually the same as in the young, although a small number of normal old people, together with a considerable proportion of those with Parkinsonism or severe intellectual impairment, have restriction of conjugate upward gaze. Nystagmus, other than a few small beats at the extreme range of lateral eye movement, is always abnormal.

The Face

It is convenient next to examine for facial *asymmetry* or *weakness*. There is often difficulty in deciding whether asymmetry of the face is due to weakness of the facial muscles on one side, or to such trivial causes as absence of dentures. Careful clinical examination is usually adequate to provide a proper diagnosis. Facial movement should be observed on voluntary effort, as on showing the teeth, and its symmetry or asymmetry noted, and also on emotional movement such as should occur following even a simple joke on the examiner's part. Weakness of the upper facial muscles may be observed from absence of the transverse brow creases, and of lack of equal burying of the eyelashes on eye closure. Weakness of the lower facial muscles may be confirmed by demonstration of weakness of the platysma. This is tested at the same time as power in the sternomastoid muscles by asking the patient to lift his head off the pillow against resistance from the examiner's hand. The fibres of the platysma are almost always easily visible under the thin skin of the elderly neck. Whether the fibres contract symmetrically or not can easily be determined.* Bilateral and symmetrical facial weakness may give rise to difficulties, but should be suspected when there is other evidence of bulbar

* One of us was taught this valuable and simple sign by the late Dr Philip Bedford; we have not seen it described elsewhere.

dysfunction, or a flat and expressionless face without other evidence of Parkinsonism.

Examination of the muscles supplied by the fifth nerve is relatively rarely helpful, but four important reflexes should be remembered on examination of the face. These are the corneal reflex, the glabellar tap, the jaw jerk, and the snout reflex. The *corneal reflex* should be elicited with a wisp of cotton wool applied gently to the cornea. It is as brisk in the elderly as in the young, and is abolished unilaterally by lesions of the fifth nerve, of the seventh nerve, and is also not infrequently reduced in upper motor neurone lesions of the face. The *glabellar tap* should always be elicited by standing behind the patient with the tapping finger coming over the patient's forehead. It is sometimes taught that this sign only occurs in patients with Parkinsonism. This is undoubtedly untrue, since it is often present in elderly patients with generalized brain disease and severe intellectual impairment, and is occasionally encountered in otherwise normal old people. The *jaw jerk* may be difficult to evaluate, particularly in patients who have no teeth, since movement of the teeth seen through the half open lips is the most simple method of ensuring that it is the jaw jerk that is being observed and not a snout reflex. The *snout reflex* may be elicited by a tap over the lower lip as well as over the upper lip. When the reflex is present there is contraction of the orbicularis oris on the same side, and protrusion of the lips. It is then not infrequently accompanied by a sucking reflex: the lips will protrude and close round a finger put between them.

The Ear

Deafness, like poor vision, is frequently accepted by elderly people as an inevitable and irremediable part of ageing. This may be so, but wax in the ears is not an infrequent cause of deafness in the elderly, while hearing aids, although admittedly far from perfect, can greatly improve hearing if properly used. The important parts of the history of failing hearing are its duration, whether there have been any sudden episodes of deterioration, and whether or not tinnitus is present.

Examination of the ears should include inspection for the presence of wax, and a view of the ear drum, to exclude gross middle ear disease perhaps with a perforation of the drum. If neither of these is present, then deafness is almost certain to be due to degenerative changes in the cochlea, and a hearing aid will be necessary. No patient should be denied expert ENT advice simply on account of age.

Speech

The history alone should never be regarded as adequate to make a diagnosis of a *disorder of speech.* Systematic examination of speech is always necessary, though many relatives of patients with disorders of speech, and some elderly patients themselves, can distinguish at least between disorders of phonation and articulation, when speech seems soft or slurred, but the words themselves are correct and in correct sequences, and disorders of dysphasic type, in which the words themselves are incorrect, and the sentences and syntax also disordered. As at any age, it is important to know whether patients are right- or left-handed. It must be remembered that the present generation of elderly patients frequently had left-handedness corrected at school, and were made to write right-handed. If so, they may consider themselves to be right-handed, but will still usually know which is their most useful hand. It may also be useful to enquire whether or not there are left-handed people in the patient's family.

In examining speech it is necessary to consider separately the voice, articulation, and language function. It is vital to distinguish between dysphonia, dysarthria, and dysphasia, and between dysphasia and confusion. The importance of these distinctions lies in the value of each phenomenon as a localizing sign, in the existence of other important disorders which may accompany the disorder of speech, and in their prognosis. Thus disorders of phonation imply lesions of the larynx or of the respiratory musculature as a whole, disorders of articulation are not infrequently associated with disorders of swallowing, and dysphasia must be distinguished from confusion because the former, by itself, is a sign of focal brain disease, and the latter of general brain disease. It is therefore necessary to listen both to the sounds and the sense of the patient's speech.

It is usually quite simple to note the hoarse or husky voice of a structural or neurological lesion of the larynx, and the irregular emphasis on syllables characteristic of the ataxic dysarthria of cerebellar disorders. It is not difficult to pick up the soft voice, monotonous pitch, and somewhat slurred and often rapid speech of the patient with Parkinsonism, and to differentiate this from the monotonous but harsh and nasal speech of pseudobulbar palsy.

Absence of teeth is a common and simple cause of difficulty with articulation in elderly people, but both the patient and his relatives will know that his speech is normal for him when he has not got his teeth in. Regional accents may also cause difficulty, but relatively brief experience in any one place combined with an attentive ear should be sufficient to make this problem much less obtrusive.

Expressive dysphasia should be tested for in the usual way by asking the patient to name common objects. These may come from the examiner's pocket or be around a bed in hospital or around the room at home. It is important before beginning to be sure that the patient's hearing and vision are adequate for him to have comprehended what is being asked of him and to be able to see the objects he is being asked to name. If a series of objects is shown in rapid succession, it is possible to pick up the least detectable degree of nominal dysphasia. It is also common to provoke perseveration in dysphasic patients. Receptive dysphasia should be tested by noting the response to simple verbal commands, and to selection of objects from a group placed in front of the patient. If there is still doubt, the patient's ability to read and write should be examined, though it must never be forgotten that there is still a small number of elderly people who are illiterate because elementary schooling came after their time as children. They are often most distressed to have this deficiency revealed.

The Mouth

Examination of the mouth should include inspection of *the teeth* (if any), of the dentures, if worn and not kept in the sideboard drawer for high days and holidays, and of the gums. These will often be found to have atrophied, so leaving little bulk for dentures to be applied to. Most elderly people who retain any teeth of their own have them in extremely poor condition. It must be remembered that hypertrophy of the gums, so common in scurvy in middle age, does not occur in the edentulous.

The palate and its movements may next be examined and at the same time the tonsils or their remnants can be seen and the inside of the mouth inspected for lesions such as those of thrush. These are white, and look like small patches of curdled milk applied often to a pink and inflamed buccal mucosa. The dentures should be removed to enable inspection of the hard palate, and to detect any ulceration that may lie beneath them.

Examination of swallowing involves the simple watching of the patient swallowing a mouthful of fluid. This should always be done directly by the doctor, and never left to a nurse or other person. It is the doctor's responsibility if aspiration of fluid is provoked. The points to watch are how quickly the fluid is swallowed, how many separate acts of swallowing are needed to clear a small volume of fluid, how complete swallowing is (by noting the amount of fluid remaining in the mouth), whether there is dribbling from the mouth, and whether coughing and spluttering is provoked when the fluid goes down. This important and simple observation should always be made on any patient with a recent stroke, since any substantial degree of difficulty with swallowing will rapidly lead to a serious but preventable problem of maintenance of fluid balance, which can be prevented by appropriate measures. In addition there may be a serious risk of aspiration pneumonia.

The tongue should next be examined. Atrophy of the papillae around the sides of the tongue is common in the elderly, and is not necessarily evidence of iron deficiency or associated with a megaloblastic anaemia. Complete atrophy of the papillae of the whole of the tongue is, however, of some significance.

The colour of the tongue should be noted. Cyanosis of the tongue and of the inner or warm surface of the lips indicates arterial hypoxaemia. Cyanosis is best observed in an indirect light, and if there is doubt about its presence, this may sometimes be resolved by getting the patient to breathe oxygen for 2 or 3 minutes. If the colour of the tongue changes, cyanosis was present, since a normal arterial oxygen saturation is only very slightly affected by increasing the inspired oxygen tension.

Examination of *movements of the tongue* is important, since abnormalities in tongue movement are frequently associated with both dysarthria and dysphagia of neurological origin, and may be used to confirm the nature of these disorders. The ease with which the tongue is protruded, the distance which the tip can be protruded beyond the teeth, and the rapidity of lateral movement should all be examined, the last by asking the patient to move his tongue from side to side. The presence of fasciculation and on rare occasions of atrophy of the tongue, should also be noted at the same time. True fasciculation of the tongue is probably confined to motor neurone disease and other rare lower motor neurone lesions of the bulbar musculature. It should only be looked for when the tongue is inside the mouth, and at rest.

Examination of the muscles supplied by the eleventh cranial nerve is relatively rarely helpful, but their involvement in motor neurone disease, polymyostis, and nasopharyngeal neoplasms invading the base of the skull should be remembered.

Chapter 10
Upper Limb

In elderly patients the upper limb presents problems of diagnosis which are fewer in number but in many ways more complicated than is the case with the lower limb. The problems are fewer in number because apart from considerable rarities only the joints and the nervous system need be considered, and there are only two common symptoms–pain, and loss of function. Vascular disease, whether arterial or venous, and lymphatic disease are all rare and when present produce no substantial diagnostic problems. By contrast, the neurological problems presenting in the upper limb are in many ways very complex, and require more detailed examination for their accurate analysis than is the case with the leg.

Pain and stiffness in the fingers is probably most commonly due in elderly people to rheumatoid arthritis, since although Heberden's nodes are extremely common (and radiological evidence of osteo-arthritis of the interphalangeal joints almost universal) in the elderly they are only rarely, and then only episodically, painful. Morning stiffness is an important pointer to rheumatoid arthritis. The wrist is very rarely involved in osteo-arthritis except after a fracture near the wrist, but very commonly in rheumatoid arthritis. It must not be forgotten that rheumatoid arthritis can begin for the first time in the elderly, and may present with a sub-acute and progressive arthropathy advancing rapidly over a period of a few weeks.

The most important site of pain in the upper limb is the shoulder; the syndrome of the frozen shoulder, with severe pain, particularly at night, and gross limitation of movement, particularly of abduction, is not infrequent. Nor is true arthritis of the shoulder, resulting from degenerative changes in the joint capsule. Severe bilateral pain in the shoulders, without limitation of movement but often with local tenderness, occurs in two important and remediable disorders, polymyalgia rheumatica and giant cell arteritis.

In general pain in the upper limb resulting from joint disease is accompanied by substantial limitation of movement, and pain from other causes, in particular referred pain from the heart or very occasionally the oesophagus, will not be so accompanied. Referred cardiac pain is more common in the left arm than the right, but may affect either or both, and may on occasion be the leading symptom either of angina or of cardiac infarction. The pain is aching and unaccompanied by loss of function, and there is virtually always some pain or tightness in the chest.

Neurological disorders giving rise to loss of function are often painless, or are associated with stiffness, numbness, or paraesthesiae. Exceptions include root pain in cervical spondylosis, carcinoma of the apex of the lung, and vertebral metastases. In general, loss of function of gradual onset will be due to joint disease or to slowly progressive neurological disorders such as Parkinsonism or expanding cerebral lesions, while those of sudden onset are likely to be due to cerebrovascular disease or to a fracture. The overall pattern of involvement is also vital, in that if there are mental symptoms, weakness of the leg on the same side, and abnormality of the face, then a cerebral disorder is virtually certain. Included in loss of function is of course clumsiness of the hand, most obviously noticeable in picking up objects or in feeding, and tremor of the hand, which again produces more obvious difficulty during feeding.

Examination

Examination of the upper limb may conveniently begin by inspection of the hands at rest. *The hands* should be examined for their temperature, and the fingers for presence of clubbing, cyanosis, and Heberden's nodes. The hands of the elderly are often cool to touch, and indeed probably normally have a lower blood flow than in younger people. But very cold hands usually denote a reduced peripheral blood flow, as does cyanosis confined to the fingers; a reduced cardiac output is one cause. The contrary phenomenon of blue warm hands and pulsating fingertips, characteristic of pulmonary heart disease, is relatively rarely observed in the elderly.

Clubbing is a very sinister sign in old age, as it is almost always due to bronchial carcinoma. All other causes of true clubbing, with obliteration of the angle and the step between the nail bed and the distal phalanx, are distinctly uncommon. Chronic bronchitis by itself rarely if ever gives rise to clubbing.

Heberden's nodes are extremely common, especially in the distal interphalangeal joint of the index finger. They are rarely the cause of important symptoms and do little to establish the diagnosis of an arthritis elsewhere.

The presence of ulnar deviation should be noted, but it is most important not to diagnose rheumatoid arthritis solely on the presence of this abnormality, which in itself only indicates undue laxity of the ligaments of the metacarpophalangeal joints. It is very frequent in elderly people to see hands lying at rest with mild ulnar deviation which can be very easily corrected, and has no significance whatever. Only if ulnar deviation is accompanied by swelling of the interphalangeal joints, and other evidence of arthritis should the diagnosis of rheumatoid arthritis be considered.

The posture of the hands should be noticed, since both the so-called striatal hand, with flexion at the metacarpophalangeal joints, extension at the interphalangeal joints, and approximation of the fingers and thumb (rather as in the 'main d'accoucheur' of tetany), and other bizarre abnormalities of posture with hyperextension of the fingers, may occur with lesions in and around the basal ganglia. Tremor at rest should be looked for, and in particular, the characteristic rapid tremor of the thumb of Parkinsonism.

The backs of the hands should be inspected for the thickness of the skin and the presence of senile purpura. *Senile purpura* is very common in elderly patients in hospital, though less frequent in fit old people at home. The lesions are seen on the dorsum of the hand and on the forearm, but only very rarely above the elbow, are purple in colour, and vary from 0.5 to 2.5 cm across. Characteristically, and unlike almost all other skin lesions, they have one or more straight edges, which may meet in a right angle. This is evidence of the causal mechanism, which is tearing of capillaries unsupported by adequate collagen against shearing stresses; these stresses act as a straight line across the skin. Each lesion of senile purpura persists for some weeks, and turns from purple to brown, without going through the customary green and yellow stages seen in an ordinary bruise. This is because there is not enough collagen in the skin to allow the entry of phagocytes into the area of extravasated blood; the colour changes in a bruise are due to breakdown of haemoglobin by phagocytes. The lesions therefore end as brown patches of the same shape, size, and site as the original purpura.

Atrophic ('senile') scars are seen in the same places as senile purpura. They are white areas in the dermis, often with white strands leading from their main body like the legs of a spider. Although they do not appear to follow known injuries, they most likely represent the results of repair of tears in the thinned dermis of ageing skin. This might be expected to stretch more than that of the young, the area of disruption being filled in by avascular and therefore white fibrous tissue.

The palms should be examined for evidence of thickening of the palmar fascia and Dupuytren's contracture. Minor degrees of thickening of the palmar fascia are very common, being seen in perhaps 10 per cent of elderly men, while Dupuytren's contracture is also a frequent abnormality, which produces more unsightliness than disability, and is substantially commoner in men than women.

The thenar and hypothenar eminences should be inspected for presence of wasting, and so should the first interspace for wasting of the first dorsal interosseous muscle. There is often considerable difficulty in deciding whether or not there is true muscle wasting of the small muscles of the hand in an elderly person. The most useful points are as follows. Wasting of the small muscles may be due to general muscle wasting, when it is symmetrical and unaccompanied by weakness, and there is loss of bulk of all other muscles. If it is local in origin, then it may quite often be asymmetrical, may involve only the short adductor of the thumb and may be accompanied by definite muscle weakness.

It is convenient next to test the *range of movement of joints,* and to test for joint tenderness as each joint is examined. The range of movement of joints in elderly people is the same as in young people. Minor degrees of limitation of movement, especially perhaps of the wrist following Colles' fracture, may be quite asymptomatic and therefore unimportant. Swelling and deformity of joints will also be noted, though it must be remembered that, of the large upper limb joints, only the wrist shows swelling easily, with obliteration of the normal contours around the tendons over the flexor surface of the joint.

At the same time as the wrist and elbow are examined as joints, muscle tone may be tested for. Particular note should be taken of the intermittent or cogwheel rigidity of Parkinsonism, which may be present without tremor. This may be most readily detected at the wrist on flexion and extension, and also at the elbow, particularly on extension.

In some patients it is convenient to test for generalized muscle tenderness such as may occur in polyneuritis or inflammatory disorders of muscle, by squeezing the forearm and upper arm muscles. This may enable a diagnosis to be made in patients where on examination of the legs there is tenderness of the calves, and it is uncertain whether this is due to local venous disease or to generalized muscle or nerve disease. Similarly, generalized bone tenderness such as occurs in osteomalacia may be tested for by springing the radius and ulna.

The outstretched hands should next be examined since they provide the most satisfactory early evidence of neurological disorder in the upper limb. The hands may be either palm down or palm up, and in either case the limb should be examined for the steadiness with which it can be held in one position with the eyes shut. Drifting or falling away of the limb are excellent signs of pyramidal tract disease and of sensory loss. If the hands are held palm downwards drift and falling away at the wrist will be seen, and if palm upwards a tendency to pronation of the hand and forearm.

It is usually possible to distinguish without undue difficulty between the five kinds of *tremor* commonly encountered in the elderly. These are the exaggerated physiological tremor of anxiety or hyperthyroidism, Parkinsonian tremor, cerebellar tremor, so-called senile or essential tremor, and least common of all, the so-called metabolic tremor encountered in chronic hepatic and respiratory failure.

The tremor of anxiety is fine, rapid (10 to 12 per second), usually irregular and variable, increased by action and reduced by relaxation, and often accompanied by the appropriate mood and talk, and sometimes by twitching of the face and undue sweating.

The tremor of Parkinsonism is slower (2 to 5 per second), regular, fine or coarse, occurs at rest and is temporarily inhibited by movement. It characteristically involves flexion of the fingers and thumb (pill-rolling), and is accompanied by rigidity, the cogwheel phenomenon, and bradykinesia.

Cerebellar tremor has a variable rate, is evident only on movement (most obviously on the finger-nose-finger test), and is accompanied by dysmetria, which is seen and felt on rapid patting movements; the pats are of unequal force and do not all arrive at the same point. There is usually hypotonia and sometimes nystagmus.

So-called 'senile' or essential tremor is common. The tremor has a rate of about 3 to 7 per second, is often coarser than that of Parkinsonism in the hands, and usually involves the jaw, and sometimes the tongue or indeed the whole head. It disappears completely on full relaxation, and is classically relieved by alcohol. It is not accompanied by rigidity, bradykinesia, or the other manifestations of Parkinsonism, nor by any substantial degree of disability. The tremor often comes on in middle life, and progresses slowly if at all, whereas that of Parkinsonism will often only have been present for a year or two before disability is considerable. So-called senile tremor is frequently familial, and there is then a history of similar tremor in other members of the family, sometimes in several successive generations. The distinction between senile tremor and that of Parkinsonism is extremely important, since if Parkinsonian tremor is diagnosed there is a high likelihood that the patient will be given drugs such as benzhexol or levodopa, which may produce side effects, without any benefit whatever to senile tremor.

The patient with metabolic tremor is obviously ill, and the tremor is of the so-called flapping type. There is sudden loss of postural fixation at the wrist when the hands are outstretched, so that the wrist suddenly drops, and then returns to its original position. Particularly perhaps in patients where the tremor is due to respiratory failure, there may also be irregular jerking movements, especially of the little finger when the hands are at rest. Patients whose metabolic tremor is due to chronic hepatic disease will have other evidence of chronic hepatic failure such as spider naevi, pigmentation, and usually a hard and easily palpable liver. Those with chronic respiratory failure will have cyanosis, tachycardia, and almost always evidence of severe airways obstruction.

Muscle power should be examined in the usual way in all muscle groups and evidence of muscle weakness accepted in relation to the obvious muscle bulk. At all times the muscles in one arm or hand should be compared with those of the other, allowance being made for the normally slightly greater power of the dominant arm (i.e. the right in a right-handed person). It is convenient to test the small hand muscles (by spreading the fingers), adduction of the thumb, flexion and extension of the fingers, wrist and elbow, and abduction at the shoulder.

It is always important to establish the overall pattern of muscular weakness, as this is often diagnostic. Thus the distal weakness of flexors and extensors alike seen in peripheral neuropathy contrasts with the predominantly proximal weakness of primary disorders of muscle. Weakness due to pyramidal tract disease is also predominantly distal, but affects extensors more than flexors, so that the first movements involved are those of extension of the fingers and wrist. These patterns need to be taken into account together with their accompanying patterns of reflex and sensory change.

Akinesia may be most easily tested for by examining fine finger movements like those of piano-playing. The range and speed of these movements may be impaired in disorders of the pyrimidal tract and cerebellum but in the absence of these, impairment is a most valuable sign of Parkinsonism.

One interesting abnormality sometimes seen in thin, elderly men is *rupture of the long head of the biceps.* This is apparent when elbow flexion is conducted against resistance. The belly of the muscle then moves downwards towards the elbow instead of remaining in the middle of the upper arm, or tending to move upwards towards the shoulder. The condition is due to fraying and eventual rupture of the tendon of the long head of the biceps as it passes over the head of the humerus. It is always asymptomatic, and indeed little more than a curiosity.

The reflexes should be examined in the usual way, and all three main reflexes in the upper limb will be expected to be present in neurologically normal elderly people. When the reflexes are pathologically brisk, a brisk supinator jerk may be made obvious by the occurrence of a noticeable component of finger reflexion in addition to flexion of the elbow.

One frequent pattern of reflex abnormality which requires to be recognized is that caused by lesions of the fifth and sixth cervical roots, due to cervical spondylosis with or without myelopathy. When this is present the biceps jerk and the elbow-flexion component of the supinator jerk will be diminished or absent, and the finger flexion component of the supinator jerk and the triceps jerk will both be normal or brisk. This pattern indicates a lower motor neurone lesion at the level of C5–6, with resulting reduction in the reflexes (biceps and half the supinator jerk) for which these segments are responsible, and an upper motor neurone lesion with increased jerks (finger flexion component of the supinator and triceps) below the level of C6. When this reflex pattern is present, it frequently illuminates the diagnosis of bilateral spasticity of the legs.

Just as there are no 'normal' abnormalities of reflexes in the upper limb in the elderly, so there are no common abnormalities of *sensation.* It is convenient to test for light touch and pin prick in the hands, and also to use paired stimuli (the patient is required to tell which hand is being touched, with his eyes shut); the sense of touch will be suppressed in the abnormal hand by the simultaneous stimulation of the opposite normal hand. This test can only be performed if routine testing shows the presence of normal touch sense in the affected limb. Such suppression is frequent in hemiparetic upper limbs and is a valuable sign of minor degrees of cortical damage.

One further very important and simple sensory test for muscle-joint position sense requires to be carried out in all patients with suspicion of a cortical or sub-cortical lesion involving the upper limb. A convenient method of testing this aspect of sensation is to hold the affected limb by the sleeve, so as not to provide any gross cutaneous sensory clues, and ask the patient to grasp the affected thumb with the opposite hand. Once this has been demonstrated on a couple of occasions with the eyes open, then the patient should be asked to close his eyes and repeat the process. When he has let go, the affected limb is moved, and the process of catching hold of the thumb observed again. Normally the movement of the hand towards the thumb should be precise and accurate, and anything other than immediate and exact catching hold of the thumb is likely to be abnormal. In minor degrees of abnormality the patient will catch hold of the wrist, and in major degrees will either miss his hand and arm altogether, or catch hold of the elbow and climb up his forearm to the wrist and thumb. It must be remembered that if the unaffected limb is weak then there may be a minor degree of ataxia and difficulty in performing this manoeuvre. Allowance should therefore be made for this.

The abnormality demonstrated when this test is positive is part of the wider problem of neglect of hemiparetic limbs. This must be recognized at an early stage after a stroke, as it carries with it great difficulties in rehabilitation. Patients with neglect of their hemiparetic limb may fail to use the limb despite good return of power, or they may ignore all stimuli, visual, tactile, and proprioceptive, from the affected side, or they may even deny or reject the existence of the affected limbs. These abnormalities may be picked up by extensions of tests such as those for suppression of sensation, as for instance by showing that the patient regularly fails to read one half (usually the left) of a line of print, or will only draw one half of a man or a house, and cannot be persuaded to recognize his mistake.

Chapter 11
Back

The purpose of examination of the spine in an elderly patient is to diagnose and assess the significance of back pain and to decide what importance to place on the presence of any deformity.

Many elderly people complain of *pain in the back,* and as with similar symptoms in other systems, the most important single fact to discover about such a complaint is its duration. If as is often the case in women, low backache has been complained of for many years, it is clearly unlikely to have any serious cause, but the possibility of the eminently treatable condition of osteomalacia as a cause of chronic backache should always be remembered. On the other hand, pain of recent onset, or pain coming on after a fall, is much more likely to be due to a fracture or to some other and perhaps more sinister cause such as a metastatic deposit. On the other hand again, there are many benign and usually undiagnosable causes of backache in old people. It is usually possible to discover whether the pain complained of is centred on the dorsal spine, or the lumbo-dorsal junction, or low over the lower lumbar spine and sacrum. Pain in the last of these sites is the most likely to have a benign cause. Radiation of pain, the presence of pain on movement such as twisting the trunk or moving in bed, and the presence of pain on coughing should also be enquired into. All these imply a cause anatomically closely related to the vertebrae.

Severe and persistent lumbo-dorsal pain unaffected by movement or by coughing, present day and night, and often only relieved by sitting up and bending forward, should always suggest the possibility of a retroperitoneal lesion, of which pancreatic carcinoma is the commonest in the elderly.

The duration of any spinal deformity is the most important single question needing to be answered. Most of the causes of spinal deformity other than osteoporosis begin early in life, and the patient will give a story of always having had a bent or twisted back.

Examination

Examination of the spine in an elderly person is most conveniently done on sitting the patient up and asking him to lean forward. The full range of spinal movement present in the supple back of the young requires examination in the standing position. This range is usually lacking in the elderly, especially in the lumbar spine. There is thus less need to examine the spine with the patient standing.

If there is a complaint of severe back pain, simply to watch the patient turning in bed and sitting up is frequently sufficient to decide whether or not the pain is likely to be associated with definite structural disease of the vertebrae. If it is, the patient will turn in bed very awkwardly, and with an obviously stiff back, while if it is not, he will turn and sit up with relatively little difficulty.

The spine should be inspected to see if it is straight. In the obese this can be established by discovering the position of the vertebral spines by palpation of each in order. If there is more than a slight degree of kyphosis or scoliosis, then the possibility of its affecting the apparent size of the heart should be remembered. Similarly on occasions a severely scoliotic lumbar spine may produce such displacement of vertebrae that their anterior surfaces may be palpable away from the midline in the abdomen, producing a hard lateral abdominal mass. Lordosis may also greatly increase the ease with which the normal aorta can be felt; it must therefore be taken into account in the assessment of possible abdominal aortic aneurysm. If there is a kyphosis, it must be noted whether the curve is smooth, which implies either the collapse of many vertebrae or of a twisting process rather than vertebral collapse. If the curve is sharp, with definite angulation of the spine, then only one or at most two vertebrae are likely to be involved, and vertebral collapse is likely to be found at that site on X-ray.

Almost more important than the determination of the presence of a scoliosis or kyphosis, important though that is, is the presence of vertebral tenderness. This should be determined by pressure or percussion of the vertebral spines. Definite local vertebral tenderness, affecting only the vertebral spines, and not the spinal muscles, is an almost sure sign of an acute process involving those vertebrae. A recent fracture or a vertebral collapse due to metastatic or inflammatory disease are likely to be found. This is the most valuable method of determining whether or not a radiologically apparent fracture of the vertebrae is recent. It is very common to find vertebral fractures on X-ray and it is necessary to know whether or not they are recent, and could thus explain present backache.

At the same time as the spine is examined, it is convenient to examine the upper dorsal muscles for wasting, such as may affect the trapezius or scapular muscles, and also the posterior chest, and the sacrum for the presence of oedema. The level to which oedema is present should be noted, as it will fall as diuresis proceeds in the treatment of cardiac failure. Improvement can be simply assessed before the total disappearance of oedema.

Another extremely important aspect of spinal function which may be easily examined by watching the patient perform the appropriate movements is that of sitting. Here the power of the spinal musculature and of the hip flexors is being examined, and also their co-ordination in maintenance of the sitting posture. Some elderly patients with pyramidal tract disease and Parkinsonism are unable to sit unaided. Patients with unilateral pyramidal disease frequently tend to fall to the affected side. Patients with Parkinsonism tend to have difficulty in maintaining a sitting posture when they are displaced either sideways or backwards, and tend to fall backwards all of a piece, with their spines straight, their hips remaining flexed. Indeed many patients with Parkinsonism have considerably more difficulty in getting themselves from a lying to a sitting position than they do in walking. They may be able to stand from sitting and walk when standing but quite unable to sit from lying.

The examination of the *pressure points* for evidence of the effects of immobility should never be omitted. The common sites for pressure lesions to develop are over the sacrum in the midline, over the greater trochanters (in patients who lie on one side), and over the buttocks, and heels. Other sites less frequently affected are over the scapulae, over prominent vertebral spines in a kyphotic back, between the knees, and over the malleoli. The first sign of trouble is redness of the skin, which may blanch on pressure but soon regains its original colour. Then blisters develop, which over the heels are often black in colour. Disappearance of the epidermis leaves a superficial sore, which may rapidly extend down to muscle and bone, which are exposed when the necrotic slough is removed. It is vital to detect the earliest of these lesions, and to prevent development of tissue loss. Proper examination and prompt action can prevent weeks or months of unnecessary suffering.

The sacral and trochanteric sites can be easily examined with the patient lying first on one side and then the other, and the heels should be inspected with the legs.

Chapter 12
Lower Limb

The assessment of the lower limb in the elderly presents a number of difficult problems. These arise partly because there are several systems which need to be considered; signs of disease of the joints, the arteries, and the nervous system are all common in the lower limb. There may be considerable difficulty in deciding the contribution of each to the patient's particular symptoms. Further, the function of the lower limbs as a whole, that of walking, is difficult to analyse in any great detail, and it is not possible to provide precise and realistic rules for the assessment of gait. Nevertheless, an attempt can and should be made to assess at least the contribution of the particular disorders found to any abnormality of gait which may be present.

The three principal symptoms affecting the lower limb in the elderly are pain, difficulty in walking, and swelling.

When an elderly person complains of *pain in the hip or thigh,* the important points to be established are its duration, whether or not it is progressive and increasing in severity, and its relation to hip movement, in particular on sitting and walking. Pain in the thigh most commonly derives from the hip in the elderly, since true sciatica with pain in the back radiating down one or both legs is decidedly uncommon; when it occurs, it almost always represents one of a series of repeated episodes stretching back over many years. Pain of sudden onset is likely to be due to a fracture, though of course even fracture of the neck of the femur may be painless.

It is important to remember that fractured neck of femur may perhaps on occasions precede the fall which is later thought to have caused it; sudden twisting movements may perhaps be sufficient to fracture the thin bone of an elderly person. A further cause of acutely developing pain in the hip and thigh is an acute arthritis of the hip.

Slowly developing pain of many weeks or months duration is much more likely to be due to a chronic arthritic conditon such as osteo-arthritis, but a missed fracture is again also possible. Here again pain will tend to be related to movement, and may greatly limit walking.

Painful knees are extremely common in elderly people, and since many old people have clinically apparent evidence of at least minor degrees of osteo-arthritis of the knees, it is a common error not to question the attribution of such pain to arthritis of the knees. Great care is necessary before this is done, since in general only clinically and radiologically severe osteo-arthritis is an important cause of symptoms. It must always be remembered that pain from the hip can be referred to the knee, and that acutely developing pain in the knee is best attributed to disease of the knee joint itself only if there is evidence of an effusion into the joint, or of tenderness along the joint line. If present for more than a few days, such effusions are commonly accompanied by wasting of the quadriceps.

Pain and stiffness in the calves occurring on exercise is the characteristic manifestation of arterial disease in the legs. It is relatively rare for the pain to be severe, and the term 'cramp' may frequently be used instead. The most important single feature of intermittent claudication is its relatively rapid relief with rest. There is also at any one time a relatively fixed distance which the patient can walk before claudication begins. Cramp in the legs at night is a very common symptom in elderly people, which though not genuinely attributable to old age, has no very definite cause. It should not be confused with rest pain due to peripheral vascular disease, since examination of the legs should reveal either no abnormality of the arterial tree or less than critical degrees of ischaemia. Pain in the legs at night or at rest is a manifestation of severe peripheral vascular disease, usually with obvious skin changes.

Some elderly people also complain of jumping of the legs on going to sleep. This symptom is common at any age, and possibly does not increase in frequency with age. Its precise significance is unknown, but it is certainly usually more properly a subject for reassurance than for powerful pharamacological remedies.

Acutely developing pain in one calf is a common manifestation of deep venous thrombosis, while pain in the calf and perhaps more frequently in the back of the thigh may be caused by haemorrhage in muscles due to the bleeding state of scurvy. Examination will distinguish between the two.

Pain in the calves and the thighs may on occasions accompany severe varicose veins. The pain is not cramp-like but described as bursting in character, and is only to be considered significant if there is definite evidence of severe damage to the venous tree.

Pain in the feet in the elderly is most commonly due to simple lesions such as corns and bunions. It is always necessary to know whether an old person attends a chiropodist regularly, and if not, what problems there are to such attendance. Here local knowledge about the availability of home chiropody and subsidized services may be extremely valuable.

Persistent severe pain in the feet may be due to ischaemic changes, but there are then always immediately apparent clinical signs. Some old people complain of burning and paraesthesiae in the soles of the feet at night. It is usually impossible to make any convincing diagnosis, nor is treatment of any great value. The best that can be done is to give reassurance that there is no serious disease present, and in particular that the symptom does not signify impending gangrene.

When elderly people complain of *difficulty in walking,* it is extremely important to discover whether this is associated with pain, in which case a vascular or an arthritic cause is likely, or whether merely with stiffness of the legs, when a neurological cause is also possible. The distance which can be walked, and the effects of stopping walking, should be enquired into, as these will be indications of both the diagnosis and the severity of intermittent claudication. Particular enquiry must be made of difficulty in getting up out of a chair, which suggests a disorder of hip movement, and of difficulty in going up or down stairs. Enquiry should also be made of whether a walking aid or a walking stick is used, and whether such aids in fact help with walking.

The diagnosis of *oedema of the legs* in the elderly rests very much more on the physical examination than upon the history, but two points can be made. The first is that the natural history of cardiac failure is such that it is highly improbable that oedema of more than a few months duration is solely due to heart disease. The second is that cardiac oedema must affect both legs, though venous or very occasionally lymphatic obstruction may make it asymmetrical. Thus the simple question 'Was the swelling the same in both legs?' will often be enough to establish that the oedema cannot be entirely cardiac in origin.

Examination

Examination of the lower limb should be carried out in the usual way with the patient lying on a couch, but in addition it is vital always to observe the patient walking, if he is at all capable of this. Examination of the lower limb with the patient on a couch should begin with the feet. These should be inspected for corns, bunions, hallux valgus, the state of the nails, the state of the skin and the presence of hair.

The *state of the skin* is particularly important in relation to the severity of ischaemia in the legs, since with more than the mildest degrees of ischaemia the skin of the feet becomes shiny and thin, and the hair on the toes disappears. The skin of the heels should also be carefully examined for the earliest signs of pressure lesions, as described on p. 31.

The rest of the leg may then be inspected for *varicose veins,* and note made whether these are varicosities of large and identifiable veins, or the venous stars and mats so common in the legs of elderly people. The latter are dilatations of capillaries and venules; the stars are arranged, as their name implies, in a radial fashion, usually around one of the points where deep and superficial veins are in communication. The mats occur in a more irregular fashion, both over the thigh and feet and ankles. Varicose pigmentation, evidence of old ulceration, and the reticular pigmentation of the leg which follows from erythema ab igne should be noted. Any bruises will be noticed, as they are usually evidence of recent falls. The ankles should be examined for pitting in the usual way, and note made whether this is symmetrical or not. If there is a suspicion of venous thrombosis, then calf tenderness, dilatation of superficial veins on the front of the calf, and increased skin temperature over the calf itself are very valuable evidence of the presence of a recent venous occlusion. Homan's sign is considerably less frequently present.

The presence of *shortening or eversion* of the limb must always be noted, and if there is suspicion of this, it must be decided whether the shortening is at the level of the hip or below, as is evident from the degree of shortening apparent at the knee.

The *pulses* may next be examined. All four foot pulses should be identifiable, unless there is substantial oedema. Absence of one or more, or even of all four foot pulses, is not rare in the elderly, even though there are no symptoms of claudication, nor any evidence of a critical degree of ischaemia of the feet. When more than one foot pulse is absent in a limb, a temperature gradient should be searched for by running the back of the hand up and down the leg. The usual sites at which it will be found are between the lower and middle thirds of the tibia, between the upper and middle thirds, or a few inches above the knee. The first site indicates occlusion of both arteries below the knee, the second of the femoral artery in the femoral canal, and the third usually of the common iliac artery. The popliteal pulses are relatively easy to feel in the elderly, as there is little muscle or fat between the fingers and the pulsating vessel. The femoral arteries are most conveniently palpated as part of the examination of the abdomen.

Fasciculation is not infrequently observed in the calf muscles of elderly people, particularly in thin elderly men. Such fasciculation is identical to that observed in motor neurone disease, but this diagnosis, with its very serious prognostic import, should never be made in an old person when fasciculation is confined to the calves. Before this diagnosis is considered fasciculation must be demonstrated at least in the thighs and arms and usually also in the tongue.

It is convenient next to examine *the joints* and muscle tone in the legs. Each major joint should be put through as full a range of movement as is possible. It is convenient when extending and flexing the knee to have one hand over it to feel for crepitus, though this by itself is evidence only of osteo-arthritic changes in the patello-femoral joint. External and internal rotation of the hip should never be omitted; the earliest sign of hip disease, in particular osteo-arthritis, is limitation of external rotation. This is frequently found to a minor degree in asymptomatic elderly people, and only gross degrees of limitation of hip movement should therefore be accepted as evidence of osteo-arthritis severe enough to give rise to symptoms.

The examination of *tone* in the legs is difficult, but it is usually possible to detect at least gross degrees of hypertonia and hypotonia, and to distinguish stiffness of neurological origin from that due to joint disease. It is always important to compare one side with the other, though bilateral hypertonia is common enough to make this of limited value on occasions. When stiffness of the legs is due to joint disease there will be very obvious limitation of movement, and in the knees almost always gross visible external evidence of osteophyte formation, with or without an effusion.

Power in the lower limb should be examined in the usual way. Movement of the toes, plantar and dorsiflexion of the ankle, flexion and extension of the knee and flexion of the hip can be easily tested, and it is also valuable to watch the patient's ability to get out of a chair (as a test of power in the iliopsoas and quadriceps) and to stand on tiptoe (for the calf muscles). A useful simple classification of power in the lower limb is:

0 no movement;
1 a flicker of movement, but the knee is not lifted from the bed;
2 the heel can be lifted off the bed but this cannot be sustained;
3 the heel can be held off the bed for 10 sec or more;
4 power better than 3, but not normal;
5 normal power.

In patient with a recent stroke, power of grade 3 or better is needed before the leg will be capable of bearing the patient's weight. Again, as with the upper limb, common patterns should be recognized, such as the distal weakness of peripheral neuropathy and pyramidal tract lesions, and the predominantly proximal weakness of primary disorders of muscle, diabetic amytrophy, and hip disease.

Examination of the *reflexes* in the legs should be carried out in the usual way. Severe arthritis of the knees may depress or abolish the knee jerk, but if the patellar tendon is correctly located, and the examiner's finger placed over it and struck with the hammer, a reflex will usually be obtained. Under all other circumstances this reflex should be obtainable in neurologically normal old people. In patients with brisk knee jerks, it is not infrequent to see a considerable element of adduction of the hip, both on the side of the reflex and on the opposite side. This is confirmatory evidence of pathological briskness of the reflex.

The ankle jerk is often absent when the reflex is tested in the usual way with the patient lying, whether or not reinforcement is used. It may be true that the ankle jerk cannot properly be said to be absent unless it has been tested with the patient kneeling, with the ankle over the edge of a chair, with the teeth clenched, and the hands pressed firmly against a wall. Such manoeuvres are usually inappropriate in examining the elderly, and the general statement that the ankle jerks are frequently absent must be accepted.

The presence of ankle clonus is always abnormal at any age. It is important to remember that this should be tested for relatively gently.

The plantar reflexes are normally flexor in old age, and an extensor plantar always has its usual significance. It may be difficult in some elderly patients who have severe hallux valgus or other causes of disorganization of the first metatarsophalangeal joint, to tell which way the toe goes or should go. Under other circumstances there should be no difficulty, though it must be remembered that the feet should be warm.

Sensory testing in the legs is as difficult in the elderly as in the upper limb, but it is usually only necessary to demonstrate the presence of touch, vibration, and position sense, and the absence of suppression of bilateral stimuli. Just as the ankle jerk is frequently grossly depressed or absent in the elderly, it is very common for vibration sense to be absent at the ankle. Indeed both phenomena may have the same cause, the frequent presence of degenerative changes in the peripheral nerves in the legs of old people. Vibration sense should, however, be perceptible at the level of the middle of the shin; if it is absent at or above this level, then a disorder of the peripheral nerves or of the spinal cord should be considered.

Muscle-joint position sense is more difficult to test for in the legs than in the arms, but it is sometimes possible to demonstrate that a patient cannot point accurately to one foot with his eyes closed, whereas he can do so to the other. It may be possible to show that the patient cannot appreciate the direction in a lateral plane in which his foot is being moved.

Gait

All elderly people who are fit enough should be watched walking. Walking should be examined in shoes, since slippers often give rise to considerable and justifiable fear of falling, and a totally false impression of the old person's ability may be gained. It is important to note both the gait itself and the associated movement of the trunk and arms. Particular attention should be paid to the gait at the beginning of walking and to turning. It is also necessary to think specifically about whether the old person's walking looks safe or not. A grossly abnormal gait in an old person who looks safe, and a relatively minor or perhaps unclassifiable abnormality of gait which is clearly unsafe, have a quite different significance, and in many ways it is more important to recognize the second than the first. The patient should be watched climbing stairs, coming down stairs (often a more hazardous operation), and using any aid that they habitually use.

All the commonly described abnormalities of gait are seen in elderly people, together with a wide range of other abnormalities equally common, but very poorly described. It is usually possible to recognize the following

1. Abnormal elevation of the hip of the moving limb, due to a stiff hip.
2. Slighter degrees of abnormal elevation of the moving limb due to a stiff knee.
3. The waddling gait of bilateral hip disease, or proximal muscle weakness, sometimes due to osteomalacia.
4. The circumduction of a spastic hemiplegic leg, in which the foot moves in an arc of a circle during forward movement.
5. The abnormal elevation of the limb, sometimes also with a little circumduction, occurring in the presence of foot drop.
6. The scissors gait, with crossing of the feet due to adductor spasm, from bilateral pyramidal lesions, or more rarely, osteo-arthritis of the hips.
7. The apparent unequal length of steps in a person with lesser degrees of pyramidal tract disorder. The movements of the unaffected leg seem to carry the foot further than those of the affected leg. If there is substantial sensory loss, the affected leg may appear to be left behind, and the unaffected takes two or more steps.
8. The shuffling gait, with small and hesitant steps, particularly on beginning to walk and on turning, of the patient with Parkinsonism. He also frequently does not swing the arms normally.
9. The wide-based staggering gait of the person with cerebellar disease.
10. The shuffling and tottery gait with small steps (marche à petit pas) of the patient with severe diffuse brain disease, whether vascular of non-vascular, and severe intellectual impairment, may be difficult to distinguish from the gait of Parkinsonism; perhaps the most useful point is the absence of any greater difficulty in turning or starting to walk. The patient may stop after only a few steps, but this is due to a restricted attention span, not to specific difficulty in walking.

Chapter 13
Assessment of Mental State

Correct and detailed assessment of the mental state of an old person is of very great importance, since many mental disorders in old age are remediable or at least capable of improvement if properly diagnosed. When the disorder is irremediable, a full appreciation of the difficulties faced by the patient and his relatives must always be achieved. Accurate assessment is also important in elderly patients with physical disorders, since deterioration in mental state is the commonest factor limiting the possibilities of investigation or treatment of the physical condition. The attitude of the doctor to disorders of mental function in the elderly is of very great importance, because it often has a decisive influence upon the patient's relatives, and on nursing and auxiliary staff who may be involved in caring for the patient and will in the long term also affect the general public. It is clearly vital that the doctor's attitude should at all times be enlightened.

The onset of confusion or a disorder of mood or behaviour is very often the first sign of physical illness in the elderly. If the symptoms and signs of the physical illness are modified or absent, as frequently occurs, and only the mental disorder is apparent, its treatment will wait upon the detection and correction of the physical process. It is obviously also important to make a precise diagnosis of a purely mental disorder when this can lead to appropriate treatment, as in depression, or when action such as admission to hospital may be necessary, as for instance in some patients with paranoid states. In other cases the precise diagnostic label may be less important than an accurate determination of the current social competence of the old person.

Diagnostic terms which suggest a non-existent precision, or prevent logical thought, investigation and treatment, must always be avoided. Foremost among these is the term 'senile', which is in many ways emotionally loaded, and should belong, but too often does not, to a previous century. A further example is 'dementia' which, because of the connotation of irreversibility in its definition, is dangerously final.

Classification of Mental Disorders in Old Age

A clear and simple classification of mental disorders is of great assistance, since it makes for clarity of thought, and thus facilitates diagnosis and eventually treatment. The following is suggested, not because of any originality, but because it has been found to be of practical value in everyday use in geriatric practice:

1. Brain failure: acute and chronic.
2. Disorders of mood: depression.
3. Other disorders; anxiety states, paranoid states, personality disorders, etc.

In practice, acute and chronic brain failure, depression, anxiety, and paranoid states are the commonest conditions requiring diagnosis in the elderly, and other disorders are relatively uncommon and unimportant.

Brain Failure

Brain failure takes two forms, acute and chronic. *Acute brain failure* is synonymous with the terms 'delirium', 'acute confusional state', and 'toxic confusional state'. The last of these seems inappropriate when the 'toxin' (when it has been identified) is a drug or is negative, as is the case with lack of oxygen or potassium, rather than positive, such as fever or hypercapnia. Acute brain failure may be recognized when an old person previously in reasonable mental health suddenly becomes disturbed. The picture is one of confusion, restlessness, and disorientation, in a patient who looks ill, and often shows rapid fluctuations over periods of minutes in mental state, from apathy and inattention to comparative lucidity and reasonable rapport, sometimes with preservation of insight. It is as though the brain were fighting against an extracerebral disturbance. Acute brain failure is usually reversible, although this of course depends upon its precipitating cause.

By contrast, *chronic brain failure* almost always presents with initial failure of memory, especially for recent events, and gradually developing impairment and slowing of intellectual capabilities, loss of interest in the surroundings and in previous pursuits and hobbies, wandering or aimless and inappropriate behaviour, blunting of emotional responses or reduction in emotional control (leading at times to aggressive behaviour at odds with the patient's previous personality), and lack of insight. It is as though the machinery of the brain were slowly ceasing to function. Chronic brain failure may be steadily progressive (synonym 'senile psychosis', 'senile dementia'), or intermittently progressive (synonym 'arteriosclerotic psychosis', 'arteriosclerotic dementia'), or it may be reversible, as in subdural haematoma, or some cases of hypothyroidism and vitamin B_{12} deficiency.

Patients with chronic brain failure not infrequently develop superadded acute brain failure. In the absence of a clear history of slowly progressive impairment of memory etc, it may be impossible initially to distinguish the two. This is particularly perhaps the case when dehydration, electrolyte disorder, or injudicious drug therapy are responsible. Under these circumstances it is vital to act upon the assumption that the usually reversible state of acute brain failure is present, rather than the usually irreversible one of chronic brain failure. In practice, a return to a mental state little different from that before the acute illness is usual, though by no means invariable. All too often, however, an elderly person with mild intellectual impairment, which is socially entirely acceptable, is precipitated into acute brain failure, by change of environment, physical illness, accident, or surgery and is then regarded as presenting a purely psychiatric problem, for which nothing useful can be done, rather than a condition coming within the scope of everyday geriatric practice.

The analogy between acute and chronic brain failure and acute and chronic renal or respiratory failure is intentional and deliberate. It leaves the way open for more detailed classification on the basis of aetiology or pathology, if this is possible, and removes obstructions to investigation and treatment where these are appropriate.

Some causes of brain failure, both acute and chronic, are listed in Table 4. Some, such as cerebral infarction, alcoholism, and hypoglycaemia, may produce either state. At any one time irreversibility is a matter of trial and error, and must never be presumed without very good evidence, which time alone can provide.

As with all other body systems and organs, it is important to have a logical approach to the assessment of the mental state of an old person. For this purpose it is convenient to consider separately the following main aspects of mental function: consciousness, behaviour, intellectual function (including memory), and mood.

Table 4. Some Causes of Brain Failure in Old Age

1. *Structural damage to the brain:*	
e.g.	cerebral infarction, cerebral haemorrhage, cerebral tumour (primary or secondary), Alzheimer's disease, subdural haematoma.
2. *Disorders of the cerebral circulation:*	
e.g.	carotid insufficiency, systemic hypotension, congestive cardiac failure.
3. *Metabolic brain disorders:*	
e.g.	hypoxia, uraemia, dehydration, electrolyte disorder, thyroid disease, hypoglycaemia, vitamin deficiency (of vitamin B_{12} or folate).
4. *Epilepsy*	
5. *Drug toxicity:*	
e.g.	poisoning with barbiturates, phenothiazines, alcohol, digitalis, etc.

Consciousness

Methods of bedside testing of levels of consciousness do not differ in the elderly from those used in younger patients. Where the level is normal reactions to speech are rapid and correct; here allowance must be made for deafness and on occasion for receptive dysphasia.

The use of a standardized method of recording disorders of consciousness is of great value in old age. The 'Glasgow coma scale' (Table 5) is entirely practicable. The best level of response is recorded for eye opening, verbal response, and motor response. Progressive deterioration might suggest a space-occupying lesion, and progressive improvement the possibility, for instance, of recovery from an epileptiform disorder or drug intoxication.

Table 5. 'Glasgow Coma Scale'

1. *Eyes open:*	spontaneously
	to speech
	to pain
	none.
2. *Best verbal response:* (nb dysphasia)	orientated
	confused
	inappropriate words
	incomprehensible sounds
	none.
3. *Best motor response:* (usually in an arm)	obey commands
	localize pain
	flexion to pain
	extension to pain
	none.

Behaviour

It is often by observation of a patient's behaviour that the first assessment of mental state is made. The sources of information include the patient's relatives, and perhaps neighbours, and also the doctor's own direct observations.

Perhaps the simplest single question to begin consideration of behaviour is: 'How does the patient spend his time?' Does he still maintain interest in his hobbies and other daily activities, in the care of the house and in his personal appearance? Does he maintain any previous interest in current affairs, for instance by reading the newspapers, listening to the radio, or watching television? The answers to such questions must clearly be taken in relation to physical disabilities, both old and recent, but failure of normal interests is highly characteristic both of depression and of chronic brain failure.

Particular enquiry should be made of restlessness, wandering, and aggressive behaviour. Nocturnal restlessness, for instance getting up in the early hours of the morning and making tea, and aimless wandering from the house, and being unable to find the way back again, are abnormalities which greatly distress relatives and neighbours. They are characteristic of moderately severe chronic brain failure, without substantial concomitant physical disability. Aggressive behaviour, both verbal and physical, towards a spouse may be part of a pattern going back many years, but is perhaps more often evidence of a change in personality due to chronic brain failure, and is again very distressing to relatives. It is also an important indication about placement of the patient, if admission to hospital becomes necessary, since both aggressive behaviour and wandering are often much more readily controlled in a psychiatric than a geriatric ward.

Other disturbances of behaviour which relatives may mention include those resulting from hallucinations, and from obsessive tendencies (e.g., repeatedly checking that doors are locked, or gas or electricity turned off).

It is always crucial to establish as definitely as possible how long any disorder of behaviour has been present, and whether it developed relatively suddenly, or represents the end of a slowly progressive deterioration. A relatively rapid change suggests acute, and a slow change chronic brain failure, but it is important to remember that either may be due to depression.

Observations on the patient's physical appearance, demeanour, and behaviour, during interview and examination, provide very valuable information. A grossly unkempt appearance is incompatible with completely normal behaviour, though allowance must be made for physical disability and for social circumstances. Behaviour provides evidence of contact with the environment, in that activity totally unrelated to apparent needs, such as picking at the bedclothes, or random and aimless calling out, is characteristic of brain failure. Immobility, apathy, and unresponsiveness to conversation, commands, or the activities of those around the patient, should be noted, as well as the converse state of over-activity, manifest by fidgeting, hand-wringing, or constant aimless pacing up and down. Hostile, suspicious, or overtly aggressive behaviour requires particular attention, for the reasons mentioned above, and so does the response to suggestions that it ceases.

Intellectual Function and Memory

Impairment of memory and of intellectual function is the commonest single mental disorder encountered in the elderly. Assessment of its degree is essential both in the correct and complete diagnosis of mental abnormality and in the rational planning of investigation and treatment of many physical conditions, since the outcome may well be greatly affected by the mental state.

Much useful information will be derived from conversation and from the ease or difficulty with which a simple history is obtained. The coherence and credibility of the latter is likely to be much reduced if there is any degree of intellectual impairment. It is, however, common to fail to recognize the severity of intellectual impairment if the patient's personality is well preserved and good rapport with the examiner achieved. The converse error is also frequent, that of over-estimating the degree of impairment, when conversation is made difficult by inattention or retardation, due to physical disease, deafness, or depression. There is therefore much to be said for those without formal psychiatric training or experience adopting standard methods of examination of intellectual capacity and memory, though these must never entirely replace the overall clinical impression as a means of diagnosis.

We list in Table 6 a few straightforward questions which have been found in everyday practice to be valuable guides to the presence of intellectual impairment and to determination of its severity. It is important to record details of the answers given, since this can form a most useful baseline for the detection of change. The questions themselves are simple enough for previous intellectual capabilities and educational standards to be largely irrelevant. The exceptions are perhaps serial sevens, the dates of the two World Wars (particularly the Second), and the name of the Prime Minister of the day (and even more his predecessor). Those of low intelligence or educational attainments may have difficulty with serial sevens, while for the other items mentioned, some attention to current affairs is needed, and some normal old people, especially women, are not sufficiently in touch with the wider world for these questions to be useful. These simple guides are only valid if mood and attention are normal, and due allowance must always be made for difficulties in communication due to deafness or dysphasia. Occasionally visual impairment may affect results by reducing the visual cues from the examiner which are part of the process of communication.

Common patterns of abnormality include difficulty of recall of new information (the name and address), combined with inability to carry out the calculations involved in serial sevens and the most complex of the three money sums ('How many 3d. in 3/9d?'). This pattern is characteristic of relatively mild impairment of memory and intellectual function. More severe impairment is shown by inability to do the simpler money sums, uncertainty about date and place, and difficulty with remote memory. Only the severely impaired are unable to give their age, or date of birth. A further useful set of questions can relate to the names, address, and occupations of the patients' children (or siblings if childless). Only the severely impaired cannot recall the names of their children, while their addresses and occupations are usually

Table 6. A Simple Test of Memory and Intellectual Function

1.	*Recall:* (Tell the patient the name and address, and ask for it 3–5 minutes later.)	
		James Anderson, 9 Kings Road, Perth.
2.	*Remote memory:*	Place of birth? What school? Teacher's name?
3.	*Calculations:*	How many 1d. in 1/-?* How many 3d. in 1/-?* How many 3d. in 3/9d?* Serial sevens: 100–93–86–79–72
4.	*Orientation in time:*	Day of the week? Day of the month? What season? What year? Duration in hospital?
5.	*Age, Birthday:*	What age? (allow 1 year error) Year of birth? Month of birth? Day of month of birth?
6.	*Orientation for place:*	What place is this? Where is it? What sort of place?
7.	*Information:*	Name of Monarch? Name of Prime Minister? Name of his predecessor? Dates of First World War? Dates of Second World War?

* These sums may seem inappropriate since the introduction of decimal coinage. In practice, old people can still use 'the old money' correctly, and these calculations will serve for some years to come.

outside the competence of those with more than minimal impairment.

These patterns are in general very consistent, so that deviation from them can be of considerable diagnostic value. Thus correct answers to serial sevens or the most difficult money sum would suggest that inability to give the age correctly was due not to severe intellectual impairment but to inattention, however caused.

A simple classification of the severity of intellectual impairment is of value, in part because it can provide guidance to the type of care the patient is likely to require. One such classification is:

Mild impairment: there is definite impairment of memory and calculating ability; such patients are often unable to manage to live alone, and are in need of some degree of supervision.

Moderate impairment: there is in addition disorientation for time, place or person; such patients can live at home with others, but if their behaviour is disturbed, institutional care may be needed.

Severe impairment: there is in addition difficulty with self-care, in particular initially difficulty with dressing; some have also difficulty in walking, and/or incontinence of urine; such patients need devoted attention to continue to live outside hospital.

Detection of the presence and assessment of the degree of intellectual impairment should always take into account the consequences of any impairment found, as shown by the patient's behaviour. Aggression and wandering are the principal aspects of importance, since they are essentially those which determine the social acceptability or otherwise of the impairment. A moderate or severe degree of impairment in a quiet, pleasant and tractable old person requires action very different from the same degree of impairment as shown by clinical assessment, when associated with restlessness, wandering, or aggressive behaviour.

Mood

By far the commonest disorder of mood encountered in later life is depression. Its presentation can be very difficult even for the experienced observer to detect. It is often mild and represents a response to adverse factors such as isolation, bereavement, or physical illness, but it is still important to make an accurate diagnosis, so that rational therapy can be undertaken. This may involve an attempt to relieve any precipitating factor, together with the administration of appropriate drugs. The distinction between endogenous and reactive types of depression is seldom useful, or often possible, in the elderly.

The diagnosis of depression depends upon eliciting the presence of its cardinal features, such as loss of energy and interest, lack of appetite, and a gloomy and despondent outlook on life and the future, which have developed relatively recently and are unusual for the individual. Bizarre and repeated physical complaints, either in one system, usually the bowels, or varying from one system to another, are frequent, but the distinction of such hypochondriasis from the manifold organically determined physical symptoms of an older person with multiple pathology may require considerable skill. Disturbance of sleep, in particular early waking, is often present, but many old people wake early (and complain of it), so that this symptom is perhaps diagnostically less useful in old age. The diagnosis is often made during history-taking, when multiple physical symptoms and the general impression that nothing is right with the patient become apparent. Nevertheless, as is the case with intellectual impairment, it is useful to have a group of specific questions included in the examination, which can act as guides to the possible presence of depression. The following are of practical value: 'Have you lost interest in things?', 'Do you often feel lonely?', 'Do you ever feel so low that you just sit for hours on end?', 'Do you ever go to bed feeling you would not care if you never woke up?' The last question is related to more specific questions about suicidal ideas: these should never be omitted if the possibility of depression is considered.

Examination may show apathy and poverty of movement and expression, inattention and difficulty with rapport, and a dejected appearance.

The elderly patient who bursts into tears during examination may be depressed, but the possibility of the entirely different disorder of emotional incontinence should be considered. In this state, which is always associated with bilateral pyramidal tract disorder with involvement of the face ('pseudobulbar palsy'), the patient is unable to control the expression of emotion, and any stimulus, particularly if emotionally loaded, precipitates almost instantaneous weeping much more rapidly than when this is a manifestation of depression. If conversation is kept to neutral subjects and the examiner avoids any expression of emotion, such as smiling, it may be possible to establish that the patient does not feel depressed. Alternatively the patient may be asked to raise his hand if he feels cheerful, and will do so, though weeping uncontrollably. It is important to recognize this condition, partly to be able to reassure relatives that it does not signify the misery it would seem to, and partly to spare the patient treatment with antidepressant drugs, to which the condition does not respond.

The converse disorder of mood, elation, is rare in old age, but may be encountered in those with true manic-depressive illness. It must not be confused with the jubilant cheerfulness sometimes shown by the very healthy and very old. The latter have insight, and their mood is justified by their health.

Other Disorders

Three other psychiatric problems need particular consideration in the elderly: anxiety, paranoid states and personality disorders.

Anxiety and agitation are not uncommon in old age, and their significance is often difficult to evaluate. It is probably rare for a true chronic anxiety state to arise in old age. Most old people with obtrusive anxiety, whether this is appropriate, and results from rational fear of theft, injury, poverty, or physical ill-health, or is inappropriate, would seem to have been anxious middle-aged or even anxious young people. But symptoms of anxiety may be an important part of an underlying depressive illness, and are then of much more recent onset. Again, as is so often the case, the duration and mode of development of symptoms are as important as their precise nature.

Some psychiatrists consider paranoid states in the elderly to be the opposite side of the coin of depression, the abnormality of mood being turned against others rather than the self. Diagnosis is easy when gross ideas of reference and persecution by others are immediately apparent, and suspicion and hostility towards the neighbours and relatives expressed in the first few sentences of conversation. If the delusions are more restricted, and are only apparent after prolonged enquiry into physical symptoms and daily activities, then diagnosis can be difficult, but is perhaps less important. The necessity for the detection of paranoid states lies in the great disturbance they may cause, more to neighbours and the family than to the patient, and their reasonably reliable response to phenothiazine therapy.

Finally, there is no doubt that some old people, whose psychiatric state cannot be called normal, defy precise categorization. These seem mostly to be people who have shown persistent oddity of behaviour throughout their lives, have antagonized all their relatives and neighbours, and are in consequence solitary, isolated, and difficult. They are not, however. intellectually impaired, frankly paranoid, depressed, or unduly anxious. The term 'eccentric' is as good as any to apply to them, the implication being of a disorder of personality not otherwise easily classifiable. Such people are usually not difficult to recognize, and the label (the word 'diagnosis' being inappropriate) is given by exclusion of other psychiatric disorders which might be amenable to therapy.

In summary, the simple psychiatric evaluation of the elderly must be considered as an essential part of overall assessment, and as lying within the competence of the physician, rather than entirely within the field of the trained and expert psychiatrist. History-taking orientated towards mental disorder, and systematic exploration of a relatively restricted range of common disorders, aided, where necessary and appropriate, by specific questions designed to alert the examiner to those disorders, will serve to make such an evaluation with the required degree of precision in the great majority of instances.

Chapter 14
Laboratory Investigations

Laboratory investigations are essential for the accurate diagnosis of a large number of eminently treatable conditions in the elderly. In general, all investigations thought appropriate should be carried out, and certainly no elderly patient should be denied the opportunity of a diagnosis by laboratory investigations on account of age alone. However, a balance must always be struck between the wish for certainty and the practical utility of the diagnosis being sought. There may be little point in fully investigating an elderly patient with severe chronic brain failure, because many of the conditions diagnosed would be irrelevant when set against the patient's general state. Lack of co-operation, again often due to brain failure, may preclude certain investigations, particularly radiological studies.

Proper interpretation of the results of laboratory investigations demands a knowledge both of the normal values encountered in old age, and of the numerous factors which may produce misleading results. If an abnormal value or finding is mistakenly considered normal for the patient's age, the opportunity for correct diagnosis may be missed. Conversely if a value normal for the patient's age is considered abnormal, unnecessary further investigations may be undertaken, or incorrect diagnosis lead to inappropriate treatment.

In the elderly normal values for most *haematological investigations* are identical to those long-established for the

Table 7. Normal Values for Haematological Tests in Old Age

Haemoglobin (Hb)	M > 12 g/dl F > 11.5 g/dl
Packed cell volume (PCV)	35–54 dl/dl
Mean corpuscular volume (MCV)	< 105 fl
Mean corpuscular haemoglobin (MCH)	27–32 pg
Mean corpuscular haemoglobin concentration (MCHC)	32–34 g/dl
White cell count * (WBC)	3–9 × 10^9/1 (3–9000/mm^3)
Polymorphs	1.8–6.5 × 10^9/1 (1800–6500/mm^3)
Lymphocytes*	0.7–3.5 × 10^9/1 (700–3500/mm^3)
Platelet count	150–300 × 10^9/1 (150–300,000/mm^3)
Erythrocyte sedimentation rate* (ESR)	< 35mm/hr
Total iron-binding capacity (TIBC)	47–72 μmol/l (260–400 μg/100ml)
Serum iron (Fe)	> 9 μmol/l (750 μg/100 ml)
Iron-binding saturation	> 16%
Serum B_{12}	> 140 ng/l
Serum folate*	> 1.5 μg/l

* Values differ from those in middle age.

young (Table 7). There is a minor decline in mean haemoglobin concentration with age, but in either sex, a value below 12 g/dl should be regarded as indicating anaemia, and therefore a need for further investigation. However, many elderly women have values between 11.5 and 11.9 g/dl for no apparent reason, and it is likely that in them the haemoglobin concentration can be regarded as normal. The blood film and standard haematological indices do not vary with age, but macrocytosis (a mean corpuscular volume over 105 fl) should always be further investigated, as a remediable deficiency of vitamin B_{12} or folate is likely.

Table 8. Range of Normal Values for Some Biochemical Measurements in Old Age

		SI units		*Traditional units*	
Na^+		135 – 147	mmol/l	135 – 147	m-equiv./l
K^+		3.6 – 5.2	mmol/l	3.6 – 5.2	m-equiv./l
Cl^-		96 – 108	mmol/l	96 – 108	m-equiv./l
HCO_3^-		19 – 31	mmol/l	19 – 31	m-equiv./l
Ca^{2+}*	M	2.2 – 2.6	mmol/l	8.5 – 10.5	mg/100ml
	F	2.2 – 2.7	mmol/l	8.4 – 11.2	mg/100ml
Mg^{2+}		0.62 – 1.02	mmol/l	1.5 – 2.5	mg/100ml
$PO_4{}^{2-}$*	M	0.67 – 1.31	mmol/l	2.08 – 4.04	mg/100ml
	F	0.71 – 1.47	mmol/l	2.19 – 4.59	mg/100ml
Urea*	M	4 – 11	mmol/l	25 – 65	mg/100ml
	F	4 – 10	mmol/l	22 – 60	mg/100ml
Creatinine*	M	60 – 170	μmol/l	0.7 – 1.8	mg/100ml
	F	40 – 170	μmol/l	0.4 – 1.8	mg/100ml
Bilirubin	M	5 – 26	μmol/l	0.3 – 1.5	mg/100ml
	F	4 – 20	μmol/l	0.3 – 1.2	mg/100ml
Protein total:		61 – 81	g/l	6.1 – 8.1	g/100 ml
Albumin		33 – 49	g/l	3.3 – 4.9	g/100 ml
Globulin		22 – 42	g/l	2.2 – 4.2	g/100 ml
Cholesterol*	M	4 – 9	μmol/l	170 – 340	mg/100ml
	F	4 – 11	μmol/l	180 – 435	mg/100ml
Urate*	M	0.18 – 0.47	mmol/l	3.1 – 7.9	mg/100ml
	F	0.13 – 0.46	mmol/l	2.1 – 7.7	mg/100ml
Alkaline phosphatase*		<150	IU/l	<25	KAU

* Values differ from those in middle age.

The iron binding saturation is the most valuable index of iron deficiency, since values of 16 per cent or less are not associated with more than traces of iron in the bone marrow. Serum B_{12} concentrations below 140 ng/l. indicate vitamin B_{12} deficiency as a cause of megaloblastic anaemia, but values in the range 100–140 ng/l. are often encountered in the absence of anaemia, macrocytosis, or neurological disorder. Similarly serum folate levels as low as 1.5 μg/l.

are often found in fit old people, and to indicate true folate deficiency values below this level are necessary.

The white blood count tends to fall with age, mainly because of a reduction in lymphocyte count (Table 8). The erythrocyte sedimentation rate (ESR) rises with age, and values of up to 35–40 mm/hr may have no apparent cause. The finding of an isolated elevation of the ESR is best followed by repetition after a week or two; if it has fallen to normal, much alarm, and often many further expensive and inconvenient investigations, will have been avoided.

The normal range of a large number of standard *biochemical tests* is unaffected by age (Table 8). In particular, the serum potassium concentration is not reduced in fit old people, and that of serum albumin only marginally, though both often fall as a result of disease or drugs.

Other tests do show differences in old age. The ranges for serum urea, serum creatinine, and uric acid are higher in older people, and there are sex differences of clinical significance. The range for serum cholesterol is considerably wider in the elderly than in the young, and high values are not necessarily associated with ischaemic heart disease or with hypothyroidism. They cannot therefore be relied upon in the diagnosis of the latter important condition. The range for serum calcium is somewhat higher in old people, particularly women, than in the young. Values up to 11 mg/100 ml (2.7 mmol/l.) may be found in fit old women.

The normal range of serum alkaline phosphatase has not been clearly defined for the elderly, because Paget's disease, and, especially in elderly women, biochemical osteomalacia is often present. It is probably best to regard values of over 25 KAU/100 ml (150 IU/l.) as in need of further investigation. In sick old people, metastatic liver disease is a fairly common cause for a raised alkaline phosphatase as an isolated finding, and measurement of its isoenzymes is of value in distinguishing bone and liver as sources of the high levels. Normal values for serum acid phosphatase, both total and tartrate-labile, are unchanged in old age. It has been shown that they do not rise significantly following rectal examination; there is thus now no need to take this point into account.

The interpretation of *thyroid function* tests in the elderly is often difficult, both for biological reasons and because of the variety of tests available and conflicting expert views on their significance. The most valuable are serum T3 and T4 levels, though even these suffer from difficulties of interpretation, low values being not infrequently found in sick old people whose thyroid function is normal. The free thyroxine index is preferable, and normal values lie in the range 0.58 – 1.24. Serum TSH (thyroid stimulating hormone) measurements are of value in the diagnosis of hypothyroidism, since in primary thyroid failure the levels are always raised, often considerably.

The *diagnosis of diabetes* in old age can be difficult, but it is reasonable to regard random blood glucose levels below 150 mg/100 ml (7 mmol/l.) as normal, and those over 200 mg/100 ml (11 mmol/l.) as indicating diabetes. Intermediate values are best viewed in the light of symptoms, a repeated random value, or a fasting value. Here levels over 130 mg/100 ml (6 mmol/l.) may be regarded as diagnostic of diabetes. Glucose tolerance tests often only serve to increase uncertainty, though at any age a 2-hr value above 200 mg/100 ml (11 mmol/l.) can be taken as indicating diabetes, regardless of other values during the test.

Other endocrine investigations are relatively rarely called for, though a low plasma cortisol level can be an important finding in a sick elderly patient who has been on steroid therapy, and this has been withdrawn perhaps because of illness.

Examination of the urine should be part of the routine clinical examination of old people. The urine should always be tested for albumin, but it must be remembered that many significant urinary tract infections are not accompanied by proteinuria. Similarly, significant elevation of blood sugar may be present without glycosuria, because of the frequent high renal threshold for glucose. Renal glycosuria due to a lowering of threshold, does, however, occur. This variability in renal threshold for glucose necessitates caution in the diagnosis of diabetes in the elderly solely from the results of urine tests.

In addition to tests for protein and sugar, the urine should be examined microscopically for pus cells, and if possible, a quantitative bacterial count carried out. Many urinary infections in the elderly are entirely asymptomatic, and will therefore only be detected by proper examination of the urine. A raised bacterial count (over 100,000 organisms/ mm^3) has a greater significance in the presence of at least moderate pyuria; hence the necessity for examination for pus cells.

Exfoliative cytology has a considerable part to play in the diagnosis of malignant disease in old age, as the methods are less arduous for the patient than most biopsy procedures, and in many cases, provide a tissue diagnosis of an acceptable level of certainty. In the sputum, exfoliative cytology provides a simple but definitive diagnosis of bronchial carcinoma, though sputum specimens may be difficult to obtain from elderly patients with brain failure. Urine cytology is very valuable in the diagnosis of papilloma and carcinoma of the bladder, and is thus an essential investigation in elderly patients with haematuria.

Almost every sick old person requires a *chest radiograph*, and so do a large number of those who are not acutely ill. A chest X-ray will ensure that the symptoms of elderly people with chronic cough are due solely to chronic bronchitis, and that there is no focal lung lestion, in particular pulmonary tuberculosis or bronchogenic carcinoma. The importance of early diagnosis of tuberculosis cannot be overestimated, since it is now most frequently found in old men, who constitute the principal remaining reservoir of infection in the community. The diagnosis of bronchogenic carcinoma is perhaps of less importance, since active treatment is only relatively rarely necessary or desirable in the elderly, but it is obviously of extreme prognostic significance.

The principal abnormalities encountered in the lung fields on a chest X-ray do not differ in the elderly from those met in younger patients. Previous films should be diligently sought when there is difficulty in deciding whether a lesion is old or recent. The radiological appearances of the heart on the other hand are greatly affected by thoracic kyphosis and scoliosis, and the cardio-thoracic ratio is thus often unreliable as an index of heart size. Increase in length and diameter of the thoracic aorta is usual, and calcification is often visible both in the aortic knuckle and in the descending part. Calcification in costal cartilages and bronchi may be evident, particularly in elderly women. Bones visible on the chest radiograph should be studied for the pseudo-fractures of osteomalacia, and for evidence of general bone thinning.

Radiography of the long bones and spine is essential if there is any question of fracture or pseudo-fracture. The changes of osteo-arthrosis are so commonly seen in many joints, that other abnormalities may be hard to detect in their presence. However, the changes of rheumatoid arthritis can usually be made out.

Contrast studies are less often indicated than simple X-rays of the chest and bones, though barium meal and barium enema examinations should never be omitted if symptoms or signs suggest gastro-intestinal pathology. An adequate barium enema examination is especially difficult to perform in a frail elderly person, and it may be preferable to demonstrate the absence of at least gross lesions by a barium follow-through examination.

Other radiological investigations, in particular angiography, are rarely indicated in the elderly, as their hazards are considerably increased in old age, and the information they provide relatively unlikely to influence management. The same is true of most neuro-radiological investigations, with the exception of the plain skull X-ray to demonstrate pineal shift, skull fracture, and intracranial calcification, for instance in meningioma. Calcification in the carotid syphon, in the falx, and the relatively common condition of hyperostosis frontalis interna may be ignored.

Computerized tomography (the CT scan) is of particular value in the elderly, since it is a non-invasive test which can distinguish between a number of important cerebral pathologies. It can distinguish between cerebral haemorrhage and infarction, and between infarction and tumour, and can also reliably demonstrate subdural haematoma. The normal shrinkage of the brain with age over about 40 means that ventricular dilatation and widening of the sulci can be seen in old people who are mentally and neurologically entirely normal. A considerable degree of cerebral atrophy has therefore to be present before it can be reliably detected in an old person.

Table 9. Frequency of ECG Abnormalities in the Elderly

	Men (%)	*Women* (%)
Q/QS patterns	10	4
T wave changes	19	13
Left ventricular hypertrophy patterns	7	10
Right ventricular hypertrophy patterns	1	< 1
First degree heart block	2	1
Left bundle branch block	2	1
Right bundle branch block	3	1
Frequent ectopic beats (over one in ten)	4	3
Atrial fibrillation*	2	2

* 5% over age 75.

There are no normal abnormalities of the *electrocardiogram* in old age, and apart from left axis deviation, all abnormalities must bear the customary interpretation. The frequency of those abnormalities which are most often encountered in the elderly is shown in Table 9. Since most of them carry an increased mortality they must be regarded as significant findings, though the overall state of cardiac function remains a much more important consideration than the finding of an isolated ECG abnormality.

Other electrophysiological tests are relatively much less important, but the EEG may demonstrate focal cerebral disorder, or suggest epilepsy as a cause of episodic disturbance of consciousness. Electromyography may confirm the presence of fasciculation in motor neurone disease, and nerve conduction studies demonstrate a peripheral neuropathy or the site of an entrapment neuropathy.

The most valuable of the *isotope scanning techniques* in old age is the brain scan. A negative scan makes intracranial tumour, subdural haematoma, and intracerebral haemorrhage unlikely, though a positive scan cannot distinguish between these important pathologies, and the ability to do so is one of the principal virtues of computerized tomography. The usefulness of lung scanning in the diagnosis of pulmonary embolism in the elderly has not been clearly shown, and other scanning procedures (liver, bone) are only rarely indicated.

Ultrasound examination is of great value in the non-invasive diagnosis of intra-abdominal masses. By indicating which organ is the source of the mass, it can suggest which radiological procedure is most likely to be helpful in establishing a diagnosis. Ultrasound may clearly demonstrate the presence of hepatic metastases as a cause of enlargement of the liver, and so avoid further fruitless investigations.

Respiratory function tests are under-used in the elderly, and have considerable value in the diagnosis of dyspnoea. They require a considerable degree of patient co-operation, but unless brain failure is severe, can almost always be satisfactorily carried out if sufficient patience is available.

In a severely dyspnoeic patient, if the peak expiratory flow rate is over 250 l/min (or the FEV_1 over about 1.5 l.) the dyspnoea is almost certain to be of cardiac origin. If the peak expiratory flow rate is under 100 l/min (or the FEV_1 less than 1 l.) airways obstruction is highly likely to be at least a contributory factor in the dyspnoea. Other tests of respiratory function are seldom helpful, except for the blood gases. Hypoxia and hypercapnia retain their usual significance, and the latter in particular is an important guide to oxygen therapy.

A number of *endoscopic and biopsy procedures* are listed in Table 10. It will be seen that some may be necessary to help establish an accurate diagnosis, particularly of malignant disease, and that alternatives to others which are rarely or never indicated are also given.

The strategies for investigation in three common clinical situations in the elderly may be briefly discussed. The first of these is the old person with no symptoms, where what is desired is as complete an assessment of general health as possible. The second is the old person with vague symptoms and no clear indications as to what diagnostic procedures are called for. The third is the elderly patient admitted to hospital for any reason.

In the first situation the objective is to diagnose or exclude a relatively small range of common conditions which are readily amenable to treatment. The appropriate investigations include tests for anaemia, urinary tract infection, and diseases revealed by a chest X-ray.

In the older person with vague symptoms of ill health, whether physical or mental, the objective of the group of investigations to be undertaken is different. They are to diagnose the likely cause of the symptoms, which may be an infection, a neoplasm or an occult metabolic disorder, and the list of tests must thus be longer. In addition to a haemoglobin and blood film, a white cell count and ESR are necess-

Table 10. Endoscopic and Biopsy Procedures

Endoscopy	*May be indicated*	*Indications*
	Oesophagoscopy	Carcinoma, peptic stricture
	Sigmoidoscopy	Carcinoma, diverticular disease
	Cystoscopy	Carcinoma of the bladder, prostate
	Gastroscopy	Upper gastro-intestinal bleeding, gastric carcinoma
	Rarely indicated	*Alternatives*
	Bronchoscopy	Cytology, radiology
	Colonoscopy	Radiology
Biopsy	*May be indicated*	*Indications*
	Skin	Malignancy, pemphigus, etc.
	Lymph node	Metastases, lymphoma, etc.
	Pleura	Malignant or tuberculous effusion
	Bone	Osteomalacia
	Intracranial tumour	Uncertainty whether benign or not
	Breast lump	Uncertainty whether benign or not
	Rarely indicated	*Alternatives*
	Stomach	Radiology
	Colon	Radiology
	Liver	Clinical and biochemical findings, ultrasonography
	Kidney	Clinical and biochemical findings, radiology
	Jejunum	Faecal fat, xylose absorption, etc.
	Synovium	Radiology

ary, and examination of the urine and a chest X-ray are also mandatory, for the same reason as in the old person with no symptoms. An ECG may be called for, and the blood urea and electrolytes should be estimated. The alkaline and acid phosphatases may be of value. Difficulty not infrequently arises when only one abnormal test is found in such a list, particularly when it is non-specific. Under these circumstances, it is usually better to repeat the test after a week or two.

The routine investigations when an old person is admitted to hospital, whether with an acute illness or for instance for operation, are little different from those discussed in preceding paragraphs. An electrocardiogram is more necessary. Other investigations should be determined by such symptoms and physical signs as the patient may present.

Suggestions for Further Reading

Adams, G.F. (1977) *Essentials of Geriatric Medicine.* London: Oxford University Press.

Anderson, W.F. (1976) *Practical Management of the Elderly,* 3rd ed. Oxford: Blackwell.

Brocklehurst, J.C. (1978) *Textbook of Geriatric Medicine and Gerontology,* 2nd ed. Edinburgh: Churchill Livingstone.

Brocklehurst, J.C. and Hanley, T. (1976) *Geriatric Medicine for Students.* Edinburgh: Churchill Livingstone.

Caird, F.I., Dall, J.L.C. and Kennedy, R.D. (Eds) (1976) *Cardiology in Old Age.* New York: Plenum.

Coni, N., Davison, W. and Webster, S.J.G. (1977) *Lecture Notes on Geriatrics.* Oxford: Blackwell.

Hodkinson, H.M. (1976) *Common Symptoms of Disease in the Elderly.* Oxford: Blackwell.

Hodkinson, H.M. (1977) *Biochemical Diagnosis of the Elderly.* London: Chapman and Hall.

Isaacs, B. (1978) *Recent Advances in Geriatrics.* Edinburgh: Churchill Livingstone.

Judge, T.G. and Caird, F.I. (1977) *Drug Treatment of the Elderly Patient.* Tunbridge Wells: Pitman Medical.

Powers, J.H. (Ed.) (1968) *Surgery of Aged and Debilitated Patients.* Philadelphia: Saunders.

Pitt, B. (1974) *Psychogeriatrics.* Edinburgh: Churchill Livingstone.

Slater, E. and Roth, M. (1969) *Clinical Psychiatry,* 3rd ed., Chapter 10. London: Bailliere Tindall and Cassell.

Thomas, J.H. and Powell, D.E.B. (1971) *Blood Disorders in the Elderly.* Bristol: Wright.

Whitehead, J.M. (1974) *Psychiatric Disorders in Old Age.* Aylesbury: Harvey Miller and Medcalf.

Index